The Secret RECIPE To FEELING Great INSTANTLY!

Revealed at LAST! HAPPINESS!!

How I found All the INGREDIENTS to Forgive the Past, Look forward to tomorrow, and smile like a split watermelon!!!

Michael Guidner

THE SECRET RECIPE TO FEELING GREAT INSTANTLY!

All rights reserved. No part of this book may be reproduced by any mechanical, photographic, or electronic process, or in the form of a phonographic recording; nor may it be stored in a retrieval system, transmitted, or otherwise be copied for public or private use—other than for "fair use" as brief quotations embodied in articles and reviews without prior written permission of the publisher.

The author of this book does not dispense medical advice or prescribe the use of any technique as a form of treatment for physical or medical problems without the advice of a physician, either directly or indirectly. The intent of the author is only to offer information of a general each other to help you in your quest for emotional and spiritual well-being. In the event you use any of the information in this book for yourself, which is your constitutional right, the author and the publisher assume no responsibility for your actions.

Other Books by Michael Guidner

- **Softly, Softly Catchee Monkey**

10 EASY CONFIDENCE 'TRICKS' To Take YOU to the TOP of the MOUNTAIN!
Work, home, relationships and love. Easy and simple if you know how!

- **The Secret Recipe for BEAUTIFUL**

Inside to Out. Lovely Pretty Gorgeous. For Women ONLY!

- **The SECRET Recipe for PERFECT POSTURE**

Revealed at LAST! How from years of research I found All the INGREDIENTS to: Banish the headaches, relieve back pain, stop the tiredness, change the hunchback, create and maintain the Perfect Posture!

- **The Secret RECIPE to FEELING Great INSTANTLY!**

Revealed at LAST! How I found All the INGREDIENTS to: Forgive the Past, look forward to tomorrow, and smile like a split watermelon

NEWS FLASH! NEWS FLASH!! NEWS FLASH!!

All that worry, blame, doubt, stalling, low self-esteem and the abyss that threatens to take your happiness can be cured without pills, potions and lotions. Best of all its free!

In 'The Secret Recipe to feeling Great INSTANTLY', eminent researcher and analyst Michael Guidner outlines the notable, scientifically proven techniques that will instantly lift your mood and assist you to grow a confident, optimistic, healthier and vibrant outlook on life right now - all the INGREDIENTS you will ever need to feel GREAT.

You will learn to:

*Recognise what causes your ill feelings that of despondency, despair, anguish and dissatisfaction

*Squash negativity

*Own your mistakes

*Handle ridicule and risk

*Overpower the need to be approved

*Supercharge self confidence

*Feel your best and

Feel Great EVERYDAY!

Fresh from the voices of yesteryear is the well-worn words of advice 'work hard and become successful' or 'hard work leads to more opportunity'. The interpretation is that as we work hard, and we are more successful, only then will happiness cover us as a cloak of contentment worn at any moment on any day and anytime we desire.

Further to this it implies if we can just find that ONE thing, gain validity, admiration, respect or embrace the ego, perhaps lose weight, change the car and become more stylish the smile will never cease, the burden relieved and the noose loosened; the jollies in life a tap dance or two away on a dance card of nonstop merriment.

But recent research, of what TRULY DEFINES feeling Great, suggests that the aforementioned is not the driver but the obstacles of futile pursuits. It suggests, that instead feeling great fuels the reward system not the other way around and all that we are gifted or turn out to be are the recipients of at first being happy.

When we are optimistic, encouraging and passionate our mindset is 'infiltrated' by hormones, signals and other chemicals which compel us to participate, create, be brave, inspire, energise and buoy at home, work or socially.

This isn't a throw away statement rather one underpinned by arduous professional investigation in thinking and scholarship, engaging the smartest of minds and the humblest of humans; anecdotal and otherwise.

In the secret recipe to feeling great instantly, Michael Guidner, draws on his own research—including the last 14 years of studies and literature. Using analysis and case studies his work enlightens how we can reboot and reorganise our minds to look onwards and upwards in positivity whilst encouraging the hormonal rush which seeks to complement happiness in order to gain that spring in our step moreover that split watermelon-like smile we long for on a continual basis.

Separating real-world, reliable 'secret' codes that have stood rigorous trials and tests everywhere from the football field to the dining table, stretching around the globe, he reveals for the very first time how we can take advantage or even exploit happiness to supercharge our each and every day and make best use of our abilities.

If ever you are struggling with the world as it stands or trying to make sense and even shine in a world of compounding demands and requests, stress, and unhelpfulness, *The Secret Recipe to Feeling Great INSTANTLY* is about how to gain the paybacks of a happier and better you collectively in all those traits; mind body and spirit, that defines us, to achieve the extraordinary in ALL facets of our lives.

CONTENTS

Preface

Introduction

Chapter 1 A Greatness Story	15
Chapter 2 The Happiness Noose	25
Chapter 3 Resignation	31
Chapter 4 Show Me Wealth, Show me Happiness	37
Chapter 5 Let's Get Great	43
Chapter 6 Awareness	51
Chapter 7 Heading toward the Happy Spot	55
Chapter 8 A Great Person	61
Chapter 9 Getting the Best out of a Bad Situation	69
Chapter 10 The Crown of Greatness	73
Chapter 11 Greatness ahead –	
8 Scientific Facts to Change Your Happiness Now!	77
Chapter 12 My List of Greatness Ingredients	79

BONUS SECTION: Loving You – If You CAN'T who can?   81

Conclusion

The Secret Recipe to Feeling Great INSTANTLY!

Preface
The Happiness PUZZLE

'Hang on! Hang on! I want to do it all differently. I want to wake up every day as though life is not a burden, a noose hanging around my neck. I want to feel good...no, no hold on... great!'

There was my cry for help ...to anyone who wanted to listen.
But strangely enough only the 4 walls of my bedroom heard. The words seemed as if they pushed off the walls and then formed an eddy around my room and that moment swirled around my brain like a whirlwind almost compounding me to yell, 'I want to be happy! I want to be happy!'
Then there was an eerie silence. There was no one to tell me what happiness was, how to find it or when and where I would experience it. No one was there to tell me this piece fitted here and there to finish the happiness puzzle.

The silence remained all throughout the day from pulling myself out of bed, slapping some clothes on to my bus ride, work station and then pondering my return journey home. Nothing had changed until I turned the final stretch towards my home almost shuffling along the autumn leave lined pavement.
And then it hit me as I watched a leaf fall from the oak tree - *Change*.

This book contains practices from my happiness, and how I did it. I'm sharing it with you now for many reasons but mainly: To allow you to move on possibly from where you've been stuck or wish to move forwards. And it starts with change.
But I want to give you the skill of change from yourself. I want you to see the many, many things that may hold you still perhaps shackle and bind you to the current point in your life that stop you from enjoying all the happiness you deserve, all the unlimited, richness of pleasure that you should be and could be feeling at this point right here. And if you don't think you have any 'shackles'...perhaps this will make you think twice. You know we all are bound in some way. And every second that we deny this we are disinclined to be open to change to correcting our self notably our way of social, work and home life and changing and so the shackle binds tighter and eventually stop us from truly enjoying life and all the happiness we deserve.

When I first had the blessing of going through my down state it really allowed me to take stock and reset my values alter my perception of life and what it was supposed to give to me.

In short, I discovered life owed me nothing and I owed it everything. That moment of doubt, shame and even guilt attached to that precise moment where I wanted to be happy made me change and it was truly only when I saw that leaf fall from the oak tree that the ignition switch would soon be turned on.

Reflecting on my life up to that time and even after it my perception of trauma, tragedy, triumph and tests were met decidedly in different ways; in thinking and action. I have had the sanction of experiencing pain from death of loved ones, poor job choices, unfortunate role models, physical ailments to fractured relationships and social choices many of the rawest and hurting situations conceivable, and have seen for myself that it is probable to experience happiness irrespective.

Modern 21st century living almost insists we find our happiness in attainment of the tangible kind; presents, gifts, money, portfolios, jewellery or other stuff. Almost always the result is fleeting and disappointing in their entirety and longevity. Aside to this there are many more of us who appear happy being locked into our own world yet when faced with obstacles and hurdles surrender to discomfort, despondency and even resentment quicker than a picture by water colour gets lost in the rain. In fact, many find it hard to appreciate there is some happiness in trying situations or when it seems the world is conspiring against them (which we know it isn't).

We all seek to feel great underpinned by much happiness and rightly so. It is what universally to a person drives us to keep going, move forward and embrace tomorrow, yet there is also hurt in happiness. The antithesis of happiness hurt allows us to appreciate the amplitude and depth of happiness. Not having one is like not having a button to do up or pants; it is what holds us up. To experience happiness, we need to know what hurt was and is, and vice versa.

By reading my awakening, my expectation is that the circumstances you face now can drive you to be enthused with all the passion of happiness regardless of those obstacles, hurdles, tests, trials, request or demands. I have no doubt you will find all the magnificence and accomplishment in all of it or as I like to call it the 'wow'; that which bites you on the bum as well as pin the invisible medals of courage and gratitude upon your chest.

Life never turns out the way you planned it, but the plans always have the roadmap to happiness along the way. There maybe a few pit-stops or detours that attempt to delay or sabotage your route but that's just another life learning experience; significant in itself and a learning tool toward feeling great.

2015 for me was a year of personal mishap tests and trials and it both culminated in that day as I shuffled through the autumn leaves and was 'born again'. It creates the perfect backdrop in our pursuit to put an end to the bad day, let it drift away from our life, and make every moment count; feeling great in the interim!

Michael

THE SECRET RECIPE TO FEELING GREAT INSTANTLY!

1. A 'Greatness' Story

Feeling great, happiness, contentment, pleasure, joy, call it what you like was very mediocre for me in the year 2014. Looking back on it my day to day life was just a consistent ground hog day; more of the same with the expectation it would return this and that to me with a minimum of fuss and trouble. Sure, there was my family and I had my hobbies however work (then as an accountant) was on autopilot and treading the thin border line of boredom and banal in receipt of it being done because 'it had to be done', regularly looking onward to the close of the week and the weekend.

If I took a snapshot of life at that point it was: Business good, money good, the next social calendar invites good, marriage and kids appeared good, yet there was void which I could not quite put my finger on. Sure, there were the weekend adventures and quality time with the family but...

To be quite honest there was something which lacked the excitement and thrill of the first times; the first time doing this, doing that, buying this buying that. In short, my happiness was deficient in the performance, exhilaration or buzz that it had once had. I was not in love with all of my happiness. Work went on day by day however the goals I had set drifted off into another space somewhere else to think about and size up. I realised that the countless hours I had spent studying being examined and critiqued, amounted to a shortcoming of where I should be in that cycle of my life. To be precise a good chunk of my life was in happy land and well a good chunk wasn't.

And then the world turned

In March 2015 I got a fever which quickly morphed into a rash meandering its way from one rib head to the centre line of my body. It was raised, red and irritating prompting uneasiness, irritability and pain; it was herpes zoster or as it is commonly known ... shingles.

In the 4th week of maddening and persistent pain, and after lying in bed contemplating discomfort and why it chose me I awoke for work and yelled 'Hang on! Hang on! I want to do it all differently.... I want to be totally happy'.

It was only on the way home seeing that leaf fall from the tree that I changed which prompted the appeal that night. 'As the seasons change so shall I' I said to myself. It was THE solution, an experience that changed my perception of happiness within in my life and that which almost bellowed from me subconsciously.

As I returned home to bed tired and drained due to the nature of my aliment I questioned the changing I had to do. I was completely gone in motivation, out of contagion phase yet felt overcome or privy to something that had no right being in my life.

That night during the persistent grabbing pain I would experience preceding the all too common moan, I questioned, irritated and angry, how I would ever get the sleep of angels; a healing sleep of angels. Then vision of the leaf falling from the tree popped into my head…*Change.* When that feeling comes that makes me groan and moan I would *change* and think of those things that would make me smile and giggle.

And so, it was a moan feeling, a giggle of surprise, a groan and a smile and do you know what? When I did it the change was palpable to my mind and body - it completely disarmed the 'hurt' and amplified the 'happy'. It was an awareness of now.

When I rolled over in bed and the scabs friction against the bed sheets I felt a surge of nausea and felt the drilling ache in my chest and hips which I took it as the ignition switch to change. I thought of three to four more things that I had in my life that enriched me; my kids, my friends, laughter, the garden. Every time I felt compromised I *changed* and every time it disarmed the significance and impact of the shingles in favour of awakenings of life and the beauty it held.

Basically, what was going on was transference and it served me well as it still does. Pain would be a reminder to me and that is the way I look at it always. It would be a reminder of all things that complement happiness; truth, love and respect. That leaf falling helped me. Pain helped me.

There is nothing like authorization of being able to control, disarm and replace those concerns with visions of positivity and trust. The discomfort of my shingles made me aware of how I could change my life not completely proofing it for positivity but embracing thankfulness. In effect this ailment humbled me and made me take stock of what it was I should be grateful for. There is nothing like the sleep of angels and I indeed had one that night. Rest, acceptance and consent made pain a reminder that events do not trail blaze my future or decide my happiness.

Realistically in my happy life if anything attempts to detour the journey of awareness I think of it as reminder that there are many things to be thankful for and to not take them for granted every day.

Whether it's a sore back or shingles, the 'flu or gout, a work or traffic jam, an argument or imposition on time, think of all as reminders of how lucky you are to have the loves of your life – those giving love; helpers, friends, and that which reminds you to love, help and be a friend.

That autumn, as the leaf fell and more particularly that night, happiness became really startling; it was a surprise almost astonishment to me. And almost from that point onward and for the ensuing days and months I treasure it. Up until that point in time I believed happiness was fate and that well it couldn't be manipulated to my advantage. I was proven wrong by myself and one leaf!

Live again

That day and that night laid down the impetus for change namely to invite happiness into my life. *Change* has been the key word since then and I can truly add that every day forward for me is a happy day. I simply have learned how not to have a bad one!

Sounds far-fetched? As 2015 continued there were many more challenges and some quite a deal more intrusive then shingles. Yet amongst embezzling at my wife's work, bullying at the kid's school and loss of my father, a dog and a stolen car I found myself still having something to smile for each sunrise. I had lastly reckoned in what manner to live a completely happy life, mentally disarm what was out of my control, accept responsibility for any 'pain', adapt to what was in my control and as a result stop entertaining a run of the mill or pedestrian lifestyle. The elements of work which threatened my sanity or created a want for banal disappeared rendered to solutions I instigated. Everything was seen from a different angle like a director instructing on a movie set I saw new lighting in situations which took on new shapes and visons when I carefully considered them. And that change meant something. The results of the new me flowed into my personal space, sleep space and family life; my mind and spirit filled with appreciation. I had indeed found happiness and rest assured it was nothing tangible moreover just appreciation and slightly more for what I had.

To live in a constant state of appreciation underpins happiness. Every hurdle or trial, test or challenge invites thankfulness; for the task at hand, for the learning process toward it and the result, and, for the right to be able to find or not find a solution to it with or without help.

Happiness doesn't accept pedestrian or run of the mill it doesn't want the comfort lounge or settling for 'as is'. Further to this, statements such as 'I'm sick and tired of my job,' or 'I've had work... I just do it to pay the bills' is virtually saying, 'I will accept pedestrian ...to just plod along.'

Think of how many times you have questioned your job, relationship and life and firmly accepted and perhaps unwittingly established 'what is'.

Every single one of us deserves more, much more than we are currently enjoying. And we are capable of more, much more than we give ourselves credit for.

The world has endless challenges and we are more than up for the test although on most occasions we question our ability to cope and measure up to each request. Instead today open the arms and grasp the challenge whether that be socially, culturally, sportingly family or at work. Let's use a different frame work when we look at those requests and often demands on our time and attention. The quest is to find the worthy in each day and what better way than to give thanks for which dares us in real time.

Rarely does a change of job allow us to experience true happiness. The trick lay in becoming the director of our own movie and looking at this point in our life from a different angle; a different shot, and accordingly we will find another side to this point in time. Simply put change occurs. Change leads to a shift in values which in turn leads to gratitude which leads to happiness. As a result, there is no mediocrity or banal but worthiness! And over a period of time since that leaf fell I which I reflect upon I realise that it was all so simple to implement, i.e. to become consistently happy. The period of time went as follows:

As the seasons change my thoughts of happiness were constantly underpinned by what made me whom I am and how grateful I was for people and circumstances which came into my life. Every now and then through winter and spring I kept reminding myself of that and was so earnest in upholding my own worthiness that on one occasion on a train ride to north of NSW I reminded myself through some notes of 'why?'. It was here on my way to do a fun run around the seaside town of Port Macquarie that I asked myself, 'how come I feel like I do?'

And these are the words I place atop the notes section of my computer whenever I write which is every day and that which adorns the top headspace of my writing pad. In fact, it is that which I have neatly laminated into something as small in size as matchbox label which rests inside my wallet and which I read each and every day upon rising and at night before bed. It covers the 'ins and outs' of why I am (see '12 MY LIST of happiness ingredients). Breathing these values is what I discovered to be the cause of my pleasure and accomplishment. And just a quick tip plenty of money or a big bust or new car didn't make it! Those things maybe boundless for some, but embracing happiness doesn't rest in the hands of shiny leather, individual selfish pursuit or rather materialistic triumph.

I realised that my words explained my happiness and I expanded on them in my list. Simply they embody fulfilment.

And there were many advantages to my list. I came to the conclusion that if something I thought, said or acted upon didn't reflect my list then it wasn't anything that championed my happiness and moreover who I was. Simply put it didn't belong!

It was created for reference for satisfaction and for bravery to tick to the values of happiness. To finally place the pieces of the happiness puzzle together although never denying it requires constant adaptation and of course work. Anything else would throw the picture into disarray and would not keep me grounded when turbulence threatened or the tempest of relationship, social, cultural, sporting or employment storms swirled around. The list was my reason for happiness and was all I needed through any time.

My hope is that you do the same; create your own list. Simply put be frank don't hold back. What are your values, morals, codes of conduct, what motivates you and why you are you? And REMIND yourself every day. The result is pure HAPPINESS every day!

When I created my list I soon realised that by loving, giving and constantly growing is where true fulfilment is found and buttress happiness. Simply put I owed people, but there was more!

By my own admission I didn't realise my list would impact upon me so quickly. It effectively guided me through the most turbulent of tempests one could ever imagine. There was some innate intelligence telling me to make my list a 'given' a doctrine of sorts and I'm truly glad I did.

The seasons change
Spring came, and everything bloomed in my life. It was a time of contentment upheld by growth and stepping outside my comfort zone creating challenges and finding solutions and welcoming change. I felt this to be so unassuming moreover simple!

It was also the time of restructuring my business giving others within my company better roles, outsourcing those that couldn't be done effectively. I found that I freed up time and this restructure within my business in turn reorganised my own personal life in terms of goals and deciding my own life line; drawn toward impacting on other people's lives helping them achieve and accomplish. Personally, it allowed me the beauty of pursuing things I felt would make a much bigger impact in people's lives. And then it dawned on me to use my education from all this and illustrate it and, so I did.

My list helped me to allow happiness into my life constantly to the extent that I peeved off the naysayers with my perpetual smile especially when they themselves were downcast or unmotivated. And when someone is feeling down, sad, upset, depressed or even angry it is for a reason. Now whether my happiness upset them I doubt it yet them seeing me like this or even coming down to their 'level' wasn't going to help them either.

It simply meant a mixture of the two and that meant communication needed to be effective and that starts always with consideration and empathy highlighted by one simple communicative tool; ears to listen with.

I grappled with the consistency of my list on many occasions, yet it was brought to the test when my son contracted glandular fever and his health deteriorated noticeably. I considered means to square-up feeling as happy as he slotted into poor health and struggled with everyday customs like dressing and eating.

But it taught me a valuable lesson. I learnt that by being uplifting and contented I became a rock of support which would only fracture if I was to continually duplicate the same angst he was feeling. I would understand the situation, but it served no purpose to dwell upon it without instigating affirmative consideration and action. Bluntly there was no point to living as one with the ailment but rather there was point to consideration and action. It would dimply serve no purpose to not feel happy about my life.

I had purposely added to my list expanding upon my words that spring 2015. And it went like this – quote, 'My spin on this world is one that invites opportunities for greatness every day. I have felt the happiness every day. It had invited me into its world to embrace it …for free. There is no cost nor ongoing payment system or due diligence. There is no badge of honour for reluctance in partaking in life. The choice is mine every day to embrace its true worth. Imagine when your body is so vibrant it imbues the spirit of each day rain hail or shine and values the essence of a raindrop, a beam of sunshine, your garden, pets, friends, family, all the relationships in your life culturally to socially and everything in between? Imagine that smile that immediately creases your face when you think about the essence of life? Your mind turns willingly to others and you embrace empathy and realise all that life was and is meant to depict. You feel great!'

And ladies and gentlemen that is simply my first thoughts as I awaken each morning. Everything is more vibrant, the birds appear to sing your song, the sun shines brighter, the rain paints a picture postcard and the smell, taste, touch, sound and sight of each day lifts you not only mentally but spiritually and physically.

And when you meet people and their face sees how radiant you face is, how your body language depicts contentment and then they almost bounce off your aura it over whelms you.

And then family experiences a joy of listening to each other' day - the good things and not so good things, the way we understand and consider each day, what we learned from it; our worthiness in its context, you feel the warmth and love. Your meal tastes better and, yet you feel a desire to impart your help and consideration to help another.

And as you write some more expanding upon your points you really value that peace of mind you now own that which makes every sense heightened with gratitude for your freedom. It is a value placed on why and what makes you tick and how each and every day with its sound, feel, sights, smell and taste encourage you to document it heartened by the questions, 'how come I feel like I do?' WHY? Why do I feel like this? And that list that you started out with gets expanded and soon you have more clarity and you have created more and prolonged your happiness and as a result mentally and perhaps physically saluted each and every day with the gratitude you both deserve!

But there is something else besides. You glance into the mirror and see a different person in another place that hadn't been there before. You see adoration, beauty, forgiveness, compassion, desire, and consideration. And you see the gifts of confidence, power and peace. For that vison and all that it entails you are humbled yet thankful almost indebted. And you feel you need to bestow your peace with others allowing you and them to connect with understanding empathy, consideration and love.

And you do it, starting with your thoughts. That 'where my mind goes my future follows' and recognise that right today, 'Now is the start of action'. You aid a friend, help family, and look to serve someone with knowledge advice and / or action. Perhaps it is a simple phone call or even listening.

You give time and help others you listen earnestly to others to understand them. So not surprisingly you don't even feel tension, worry, dissatisfaction or fright for you walk your own path; that is, you are responsible for what you do and where you go. Sure, there may be some guilt, (everyone, at some stage of their life, wears self-guilt – you just don't want it to be a comfortable fit) and you adjust your thoughts and if need be replacing them with better ones.

Further to this you find yourself creating joy and confidence and you change for Life itself is ever-changing often courtesy of those who change it – a difference to others and to yourself. You realise every single day that you have a chance to be new like each dawning day, pristine, embodied by good deeds done and good words spoken. You know you attracting all the happiness you need.

And at the end of a highly dynamic, wonderful day, you welcome the love of all around; friends, associates and family. You treasure each moment with each child, each loving word, and thought. You cherish the peace. You are amazed at the wonder of life.

As the day closes and you lay back in bed and you reflect on that day you become at one with contentment all that you have dome and been given. You realise the reason for being here is that you are a good person looking to embrace challenge that rewards you with awareness, understanding, acceptance and respect and love. Strength is all this.

Can you really believe all this to be possible?
It is. It just rests within waiting for you to embrace it.

So that was my world at the time. My list, my Recipe to feeling happy and great, was and still is a great big part of it; simply, a reminder of how I changed and why and the reasons happiness came for me. My list is a reminder of the way to live. I must say that I struggled at some stages because as the world is not perfect so am I for everyone, at some stage of their life, wears self-guilt, the fact is you just don't want it to be a comfortable fit; and just as I create angst and apprehension; I create joy and confidence. I know from experience the Recipe to feeling Great instantly!

2. The Happiness Noose
Why do we make Happiness So Hard to attain?

If happiness is a universal goal, then we need to understand its cause and effect. But before we go on to the studies and definitions, we need to know why it's so important to us. Why are we so hung up on being happy?

The Benefits of Being Happy

...Is good for your well-being. Happy people have durable resistant systems i.e. stronger immunity against illness, disease and ailments and have an extended pleasure duration, than disheartened and unhappy people.

...Makes you more giving. There is a willingness to share good fortune.

...More able to combat against stress. Quicker to bounce back after shock and distress.

...Improves relationships. Most happy people have a broader and more meaningful network of friends.

...Embolden success. Happy people are more artistic, imaginative and energized at home, socially and especially at work.

...Happy people are reported to live more than 10% longer than Mr and Mrs Doom and Gloom or their cousins 'the sad sacks', increasing their lives by up to 10 years.

The recipe for Happiness is universal quest; a search for that missing ingredient. It is a human endeavour – a universal goal.

We all want to be happy, and we empathize with each other's need for it. We search for it with all our might, our thoughts and actions focused on only one goal in happiness – to be happy. The search for happiness involves deep thinking and assessment not earth-shaking neurone stimulation but valid common sense sadly which a good deal of people lacks.

Let's break it all down into some more simple and easy stuff.

Why is Happiness so difficult to attain?

Well we've discussed appreciation and its other names 'gratitude' and 'thankfulness' but there is more. It's easy to have a life of extremes; doing very little (disappointing) or over scheduling (exhausting). A healthy happy happiness sits somewhere in between balancing the emotional as well as the physical scales.

One must understand not just the cause of happiness but also the physiological and pathological effects which it can produce, and the ways in which it's adverse and self-deflating tendencies can be countered.

For the best results such simple common-sense strategies need to be combined with methods which effectively increase and enhance the natural defences against stress, which some people have in greater or lesser degree than others. The importance of reviewing, and altering where necessary your diet, exercise and rest patterns, personal attitude, as well as behavioural patterns (many of which are within our conscious control) are all features of this plan which can deflect many of the potential harmful effects upon hectic modern-day happiness.

If our passage of happiness is analysed or philosophised, then many burning questions with the same undercurrent tempt us all:

'Why is happiness so different?'

'Why is it easy for some?'

'Why is it so hard for most of us?'

The focus of why we need let the sunshine into our happiness and how we go about doing it is a dominant conversation topic. Many answers have been documented. The reality is happiness, at times, can be a burden but we must ensure the focus on happiness being a burden doesn't subtract from its true passage – life is for living with all its bits and pieces. All we need to do now is take the necessary steps to ensure we remain focused on pursuing this enjoyment and happiness.

At some stage in our lives we seem to suffer an endless bombardment of arrows that are shot at us. We seem to be the moving target. The momentum feels as though it will never cease but why does it feel so?

Maybe the answer lies in our reaction to those events which tests us all:
...Of love won and lost;

...Of illness, disease, sickness, recreational or work accidents;
...Of words left unsaid;
...Of loss of marriage, relationship, family, children and work;
...Of loss of physical or mental strength
...Of patience lost.

The definition of happiness varies according to whoever defines it:
'Your happiness has no price. It cannot be bought. It is not an app that you can download on your phones, nor will the latest update bring your freedom and grandeur in love.' – Pope Francis

Omar Khayyam, 'Be happy for this moment. This moment is your life.'

Albert Schweitzer 'Success is not the key to happiness. Happiness is the key to success. If you love what you are doing, you will be successful.'
Buddha, 'Thousands of candles can be lighted from a single candle, and the life of the candle will not be shortened. Happiness never decreases by being shared.'

But what is happiness, really? Is it that feeling when you cross the finishing line first, awarded a trophy, courted with jewels, a sexual interlude, a new car or when you love someone, and they love you back? You know it when you're happy or not, but can something so intangible really be defined and measured?

Current studies of happiness indicate have shown that there are firm needs that must be fulfilled in order to achieve this emotional state. Of course, this is enduring happiness not the fleeting endorphin rush perpetuated by a new car, diamond ring or lavish home.

In the study of Human analytics researchers agree that humans are happiest when their life involves the Wonderful 8:

1. Common-sense Choice (indulging one of the 5 senses)

2. Activity (doing what you are avid about)

3. Associations (constructing social and community networks that are important)

4. Significance (engaging with and for something which transcends physicality – i.e. emotional and spiritual awareness)

5. Deed (the completion of tasks)

6. Uncertainty (acceptance that uncertainty is not some abstract attachment to life but a natural part of life)

7. Spontaneous 'up' events (those unexpected circumstances that have some significance – short happiness)

8. Reflection of judgement imposed on our self about our overall well-being – a feeling thing.

Whatever way you define your happiness it is important to strive for longevity in happiness for as we know the excitement and euphoria of short term gifts and events (often what people aspire to) are fleeting at best.

So, with this in mind, one should aim for consistent elation. Often this is armed with a steady endorphin rush which signals a state within the mind and body of contentment and often peace. So, happiness is deeper than the quick fix and for longevity there needs to be something substantial to mental health, spiritually or emotionally, that fortifies a smile, joy and desire to involve oneself in the passage of each day, day in day out.

There is a common misconception that we should try to fix things and get happy or resolve at any cost those trying troubling occasions that threaten our calm. Sometimes we simply need to acknowledge feelings. By acknowledging feelings, we don't allow them to usurp the value of our day or compete for our undivided attention. Once you can acknowledge the feelings they won't jeopardise your day for you have already begun to route feelings that detract from happiness. And there is one thing key in all of this...the mind.

Even Confucius a Chinese philosopher, from 551 B.C – 479 B.C suggested the mind has a substantial role in attaining happiness after-all that is where the reaction to action and the initial spark of suggestion and permanence begins and fosters. He always advocated focus on social relationships and the great virtue of 'humanity': 'They must often change, who would be constant in happiness or wisdom.'

Perhaps the complete definition of happiness I like to use is 'living through the eyes of someone else'. When you can master that you have shown that you love yourself enough to be thankful, grow, change, realise life and empathise with another.

Whatever your definition of happiness maybe there are ALWAYS the underlying basis which supports a grin and gratification, and these are the same factors for rich or poor; there is no discrimination.

Where applicable some cars used to have duco described as 'weatherproof' but this expression now tends to be altered to 'weather resistant'. In making such assertive appealing statements the car manufacturers have had to assess the properties of the car, its detail, construction and cover as well as the different sorts of weather it may be subjected to and the text which underwrites when and where that resistance may falter e g. act of god storms. There are other hazards, too, facing the car duco such as aeroplane fuel expulsion, radioactivity, battery acid leak and graffiti; such 'weather' one can't really plan for in short doses. These factors can all or in part impact upon the cars duco.

In the same way we face a range of happiness factors that challenge us during the course of our lives, and it is not possible to 'happiness- proof' ourselves completely. However, we can put the necessary steps in place to increase our ability to handle those obstacles that threaten our happiness. Sometimes our responses to events will be weak yet however ineffective these responses may feel there is always a positive to be had from a negative situation which only serves to enhance our happiness further. (See chapter 9 *getting the best out of a bad situation* for more).

Variables exist not only in the nature but also in happiness unique in characteristics certain of us. Some of us are born with a strong degree of these characteristics which I call Dynamic Pliability whilst others seem to be short of this ability to readily, adapt change and even defend.

The Dynamic Pliability Factor is a combination of things, including a sense of what greatness, and those events underpinning it, truly mean. It is also the feeling that the multiple changes which occur throughout being the best we can be present challenges or opportunities rather than threats. Moreover, the Dynamic Pliability Factor aids and abets change to effectively become involved in society and the lives of others. Whilst on the surface you may sense the pliability factor is a hard badge to attain the good news is that, as with so many aspects of feeling great and experiencing happiness, these positive character building characteristics can be learned. Once learned they will NEVER leave you.

The state of your wellbeing; greatness and happiness, is the sum of the interactions between the uniqueness of you; that is your values, morals and boundaries, and the challenges and stresses of your individual environment. The latter stresses may involve job insecurity, an unstable marriage, social angst, financial drama, family strain whilst most happiness is made up of attitudes, beliefs, behaviour patterns, personality traits (the major features of the dynamic pliability factor) and deeply conditioned or nurtured traits. Add to this the importance of correct food choices, sufficient exercise and rest, life style choices as well as the benefit of mother nature in helping to reset our balance and the sum of the interactions become clearer.

If there is any amount of actual happiness proofing, then it involves taking responsibility for your life most of which involves cognitive reappraisal necessary to reassess the meaning of events.

A hurricane can cause much chaos yet in the eye of this very same hurricane there is a quiet. In life there is much chaos but in its quiet there will be moments of great love, connection, compassion, empathy and development. Many great scholars have suggested it's not the happiness that's so hard, but the living of it, the quiet, and happiness is hard because we made it so. And if we dwell upon the negativity of our existence it`s called resignation.

3. Resignation

The bullies of this world go out looking for a fight; to win a war verbally or physically. It is a void in their life compounded by poor choices, ignorance and low self-esteem and highlighted by severe unhappiness. So, what about people who aren't bullies? What do they find? And what finds its way to them?

One would suggest feeling great, contentment or happiness is knowing that they are a good person but one of the critiques of happiness that make us unhappy and strengthens the case to give up is a common everyday postulation – 'I am insignificant'. Often the everyday non-bully doesn't get noticed and doesn't receive the bouquets or plaudits for their way of life and this can cause them to question how they feel about themselves.

The bully seems to always be noticed and that give rise to concern. Soon if one tires of being consistently nice or adhering to what is considered the rules of life one may look for negativity attaching dissatisfaction to being who they are. They may struggle with maintaining their identity seeming for no reason. Is this you?

This is resignation. Simply put it means one embraces defeat and cements it firmly in life. It is by far the quickest yet most destructive force to happiness and a common default programme to activate. Quite often this occurs before starting the task at hand. Now the stone is effectively the burden of dismay, juggled constantly from hand to hand and is the most obtrusive invasion into positive thinking. Now, as the stone is held the chance to change things is lost.

Why?

The answer to this resignation lay deep within the brain and it's called Mindset.

It takes practice and persistence to change deeply ingrained thought patterns. Knowing this, ask your-self: How hard am I willing to work for happiness? For really living unhappy is far more taxing then doing all the preparation for a happy one. No one ever improved their happiness or changed others in the process with an adverse and self-deflating profile in their happiness. Your suffering is not a badge to wear on your chest as marker of bravery or valour moreover it really is one of regret and despondency. It is mindset.

Resignation means one cannot or does not want to improve their situation. In improving your situation, it doesn`t mean you have to win or be right or be noticed.

Moreover, if one assumes he/she could win, that would have been positive thinking, which has its it`s time and place. But crushing resignation is more exact and moreover basic, it doesn't require trying to convince oneself of something one should be convinced of or even capable of - it is simply not aiming up for the task ahead, whether that be physical or mental and that usually takes place as a result of a request.

The reality is people acquiesce to the staleness of some of the demands of happiness instead of favouring the work that goes into being happy. They accept the situation is hopeless when it essentially isn't. And so, the lights are turned off. Ideas go unchallenged, dealings and relationships dissolve, finances fall into disarray and children turn unbecomingly. The darkness now becomes a lonely place. There are no accomplishments in the darkness. Now the assumption that happiness is too hard and offers no enjoyment is constantly entertained.

The creation of resignation (the defeatist) and the committed emotions soon become engrained within the human essence and if repeated they the defeatist become accustomed to expecting it. Now they think of themselves as failures or also-rans and so don't expect anything dissimilar. They sabotage their happiness through repetitive acclimatizing. Now the goal is impossible. That's resignation. And the mindset behind it is almost always wrong but often durable.

Make no mistake, stumbling blocks frequent the passage of everyone but it is the response or reaction to this setback that fosters your will to move forward.

Most appliances come with guarantees; warranty against faulty parts; for a new vacuum cleaner you may get 12 months and for a new car perhaps years; a guarantee of sorts against incongruities. However, we cannot guarantee the physical parts of our life which run poorly or collect on insurance for the mind if it has trouble coping with the tests and trials modern 21st century living delivers.

We all will face a range of happiness obstacles that challenge us during the course of our lives, and it is not possible to guarantee sustained 24/7 happiness. It could never be done and never will be done. However as mentioned prior there are steps vital in dealing with unhappiness and those obstacles which may attempt to detour us from our right to be happy.

The Dynamic Pliability Factor allows us not to be affected by minor inconsistencies in our life and allows us necessary skillset to deal with that which attempts to detour us from the happy route.

Often, when we are unhealthy our outlook to happiness varies significantly. A person who struggles being overweight underweight, consistently ill or in chronic discomfort can be overcome with enough self-doubt to ignite the resentment, fright and failure which of course becomes externally generated through challenges we or others create. The term given to those challenges are erroneously and commonly called setbacks.

Explanation and analysis are the two keys to understanding the situation at hand. Setback can make you feel worse and inevitably renders you immobile. Now, you throw up the white flag; surrender.

But how does one keep from giving up?
How does one keep from surrendering to misplaced scruples?
How does one maintain the zest for happiness?
How does one seek the goal and live the dream of happiness?
The answers can be as complicated or as simple as you make it.

If one's relationship is in disarray, the way one both analyses and explains this setback will determine whether one has reached an important juncture in the relationship, or is about to light the wick of the resentment bomb.

People who analyse and can sensibly explain a setback are less likely to give up on what they need. Firstly, they recognise it as a challenge and they garnish a sense of their power and are committed to achieving contentment instead of surrendering to its opposite i.e. - discontent. If something is changeable or preventable, it makes a big difference whether one understands that it is. It is very important to accept it as a challenge and that acceptance comes from two things – analysis and explanation.

If we can analyse where our happiness wanes and why (explanation) then the necessary adjustments can be made. Is it a non-committal family member regarding appropriate aged care? Is it a clash of moral views, boundaries or codes of conduct? Is it unfair decisions at school that affect you child or implausible decisions at work that discriminate against yourself? Is it a relationship that doesn't justify time and energy due to a difference in attitude? The studies of all this indicate in some way happiness becomes drained.

From the middle of the 20th century (the early 1960's to be exact) science has involved itself in the study of what makes people happy and how people can live happier.

One result from the 75-year Grant Study of Harvard undergraduates showed significant correlation to a nurturing and loving relationship between students and their parents in real time which many years later manifested as continuing happiness. Further to this Finnish research on over seven hundred people has suggested happiness encompasses every part of our body in its significance; i.e. bottom to top! Money only provided the icing on a rather larger cake of contentment. Furthermore, there were more ingredients to the cake which espoused the greatest happiness which was further buttressed by a Harvard school of business. Their study suggested helping others financially and giving more were notable factors which created more individual happiness then if one was self-indulged.

Perhaps it is common knowledge, but relationships play a significant role in the longevity of happiness. The longer and more involved the relationship the more rewards pin personal growth and attach to self- esteem.

Spiritually some studies suggest the greater belief you have the more tendency you have to be happier. However according to studies from the University of British Columbia, 2012 religious people just like non-religious who create and have ongoing communal contact espousing the values of helping, giving, listening and communication grow happier each day. So perhaps the basic structure of empathy doesn't discriminate between religious and non-religious.

Science also suggests oxytocin plays some role in continuing happiness.
A hormone common at child birth well known as the hug drug oxytocin has an important role in happiness whilst exercise, according to scientific analysis at Bristol University in the U.K in 2008, said to increase endorphins, blood flow, diminish niggling impact of injures and create a warm post glow which nurtures the happiness factor. Bristol even emphasised prior studies on the effect of exercise on happiness after data suggested people's moods significantly improve after engaging in exercise. (UK University of Bristol, 2008)

Even the University of California in 2008, suggested from their scientific research that happiness is infectious and that just by being around smiles and laughter you can 'catch' the bug!

But hang on why is that we feel better when we go on to retail therapy?

Well latest research in from San Francisco State University, 2009 indicates it's not the gifts we buy, but the *effect* of being able to go shopping which does it.
Academics and pious thinkers often define happiness in terms of a decent life or embracing the values or ethics of a leader. Now one finds the psychological aspects far

outweigh the religious ramifications of not living a 'proper' life although perhaps the rules of religious orders and philosopher's orders are often underpinning by common-sense. Still, religious or not the science behind resignation indicates the defeat of values and an erosion of mindset. It occurs, and one truly has to be diligent in awareness.

4. Show me wealth, show me happiness

We have all had those dreams...winning the lottery, diving into truckloads of cash, the new car, the better job, a bigger house or the best partner in the world. Life couldn't get any better or any happier if we only had that...right?

And then it happens and what was intended to be the Utopia of happiness, that feeling of invincibility because we are loaded with dosh or materialistic treasures suddenly dissipates with time now a brief blimp in our own history; a brief interlude in the rhythmical melody of life's journey.

And then it dawns upon you like an early unexpected early morning ray of sunshine after a rainy night, when you finally got it, that happiness boost didn't last that long or wasn't as intense as you'd imagined, right? Why didn't that stint of happiness last longer and if it couldn't where be the long-lasting happiness we all want in life?

What is that all about?

Perhaps the answer lay within the term The Hedonic Treadmill (hedonic adaptation). The hedonic treadmill is a notion proposed by two leading psychologists, Brickman and Campbell, in the early 1970's that suggests that individuals return to a sense of happy balance regardless of what immediate experience they are involved in.

Everything in life seeks equilibrium. That is the job of nature is to restore balance; water finds its own level and temperatures do not remain constant all year; we have the seasons to help nature readjust and the animal food chain.

So, it goes when we are sick; the body seek homoeostasis; a return to balance or equilibrium and after much therapy, rest or intervention most of us return to a 'normal' state of wellness not supercharged and hopefully not depleted.

Further literature suggests there is The Happiness Set Point which refers to the inherently firm tendency for happiness that is responsible for about 50% of the differences between you and everyone else. That is, you are genetically programmed for this set point which determines more than half of the way you will respond to 'happiness'!

In her book 'The How of Happiness' researcher Sonja Lyubomirsky says that: If you struggle with a low set point, meaning, you tend to gravitate towards despondency or depression, don't be so hard on yourself, to an extent you're dealing with a stacked deck.

However, remember this; the stacked deck still contains some aces which as we all know in playing cards can be the winning cards. So, in light of what Lyubomirsky suggests cognitive brain training can turn the default programmes slanted towards negativity in favour of positivity. It may be a case of the glass half full instead of half empty which has much credence in fortifying thought and action.

Therefore, conditioning in spite of genetic predisposition for the sadder side of life can be overcome. It is not a 'given' to be passed through the genetic course.

As I hinted on earlier, recent research indicates regarding the happiness we have a default button to which we return regardless of the euphoria or dissatisfaction /despondency we may experience. It is a return to equilibrium or as Lyubomirsky suggested a set point. Simply put if you get married, move into a new house, get a promotion, lose a job or suffer an accident, for example, after a certain period of time you're likely to return to your set point'.

Sure, there is the ignition of the pleasure dome after or during an exciting event but soon after the balance returns.

Studies by Brickman and Campbell proposed that our sensory structure returns to the level prior to the event, after some time. This conclusion turned out to be essential for researchers learning about happiness for it emboldens further insights and analysis of the recipe for happiness.

One further study of the 'treadmill' involved analysis of people who won the lottery and para and quadriplegic victims. In their published essay in 1987, Brickman, Coates, & Janoff-Bulman 'Lottery winners and accident victims: is happiness relative?' discussed the various factors and setting which maybe the ingredients to the happiness. The study noted that both groups were dealt large emotional strikes with respective reactions of happiness and despondency, but effects revealed soon after that there 'set point' or point of equilibrium returned. That is, they returned to what happiness they had prior to each incident after a period of time.

In the original treadmill theory however, the authors (Brickman and Campbell) proposed that people immediately react to good and bad events but in a short time return to neutrality. But further research led by Ed Diener went a little further. His study suggested the following:

I. The set point is not neutral

ii. The set point is individualized

iii. We have multiple set points

iv. Happiness can change

v. Individual differences in adaptation

i. After reviewing the studies Diener & Diener found that approximately three quarters of the samples reported a balance affect (positive and adverse and self-deflating moods and emotions) above neutral. That is the set point favours happiness overall instead of gloom and doom and this is significant. It simply means the mind body and spirt seek contentment over misery on a constant basis day in day out.

The studies further suggested that even in varied populaces including remote African tribes the well-being level was above neutral.

ii. The set point is individualized

Studies suggest everyone's' set point is different or personalised. Research indicates personality traits, headed obviously by opinion, moral code and values, have a big say in things and further to this health and well-being had its footprints in how one treats their mind and body.

iii. We have multiple set points

Recent work by Lucas, Diener and Suh reveals happiness is a derivative of multiple different dynamics and is not interconnected.

For example, on one instance, you could have both constructive and optimistic, and, destructive and pessimistic emotions in decline but approval on the rise, the notion being that different feelings can move independent of each other. Rather obtuse but nevertheless debatable.

iv. Happiness can change

One of the conclusions often drawn from the first study is that no matter what we do we can't affect much change into our long-term level of well-being and life satisfaction.

Fujita and Diener designed a longitudinal study that examined changes in the baseline level of well-being over a period of 17 years in a large sample group of Germans. They wanted to know whether happiness can be changed. They found that even though there was significant stability in the happiness assessments, 24% of participants did experience significant change to their happiness level. So, it seems that long lasting change is possible.

Thus, your circumstances often come under voluntary control and so the result of that change is up to you – i.e. happiness can be changed.

v. Individual differences in adaptation

Another allegation from the original theory is that adaptation to events happen quite the same way to everyone.

We all know we respond to requests and demands on our time in different ways and that in it lay the platform for prospect of happiness. There is one strong demand on us as individuals and that is when we choose to unite with a partner sharing concerns and values.

Lessons into adapting to change within marriage forecast that the happiest folks would respond more intensely to positive events. But the results showed otherwise, that less satisfied individuals were more likely to benefit from marriage in the long term.

The above almost emphasises the aces in the stacked deck of cards that all of us will get to play and utilise effectively if we desire.

Are we on the treadmill forever?

Most studies agree that gratitude, communal celebration and giving are integral in adjusting the treadmill. Most of this can start with awareness; a meditative technique to train our mind into what it is that defines happiness and what detracts from it.

Happy people know how to react to an act imposed upon them, they know how to dismantle the futility of some situations and disarm the stress attached to those situations they have no control over (which is most), whilst unhappy people, by difference, indulge the adverse aspects of progressive events or entertain constantly how life; events, society, and morale, was better before. In turn they almost sense a doom and gloom often infiltrated by defence mechanisms in the form of such statements as, 'It always happen to me…' an attitude that confirms their reaction to events which more often than not dwells on impact and the burden attached.

One must remember to be aware of one's initial reaction to situations and take stock and view the situation as someone looking upon it as bystander. Often only then can one get a real sense of what is needed and what is not. To propel our positivity towards happiness revisit times when everything clicked and replace our negativity with that which we felt proud and joyful.

Therefore, in summary even though the 'set point' may be something worth considering there is the undeniable ability of the individual in adaptation processes across events, considering upbringing, genetics and personalised traits of morals, values and codes of conduct.

THE SECRET RECIPE TO FEELING GREAT INSTANTLY!

5. Let's Get Great!

Where potentially do we fall down, when it comes to being happy and feeling great?
Firstly, it's important to understand we want as prerequisite principles to justify ourselves. However, more often than not, laying down our own set of principles (rules and codes) can be difficult. Principally we want all our ideals to be met and when they aren't how on earth we can ever manage happiness or feel like we are on top of the moon? When everything falls outside our boundary lines and we feel violated when it comes to values, morals, rules and codes then happiness eludes us.

We envision 'idyllic' situations –as we do the opposed of those visualisations. We associate the present and all that it embraces at this point with those visions. Sometimes this is what holds us back from happiness – the expectation that things should be and should have been better.

The smile creases our face and warms our heart when we sense ourselves reaching, or even just stepping nearer our idealized visions. However, if we don't sense ourselves reaching or even just approaching these visions then our pride; through which we work, play, relate and seek gratification; become community aware, determine our journey and learn, fails to be united. Now, we have failed to reach our own expectations. To be happy is to feel oneself moving along our expectation line to the rewards picketed along each line post toward the 'bounty' at the end.

Expectations shift as we move through life frequently. Those expectations are modified or lowered allowing our happiness to be altered in the interim. The shift within life may simply be related to wisdom or maturity and often a combination of both. Often the obstacles that confront us and cause us to hesitate or stop at each expectation line post reticent to take the next step and meet our expectations are the ones where we compare ourselves to what society expects of us; our class or state of affairs. Sometimes, that is a bit like 'keeping up with the Joneses' whereby we seek to accomplish tasks or have things in order to maintain some sort of pecking order incidentally only 'important' to ourselves.

Yet because our emotions feature expectations and having them met, then unhappiness entails 'the miss's or feelings of loss accompanied by self-ridicule, denial and impending despondency.
Further still unhappiness also calls into account past events, such as misplaced words or actions or a dishonour that can never be remedied.

Often society has a lot to answer for as it encourages incongruence in goal setting and attention getting which plays on people's inferiorities. This effectively erodes their rights to live unaffected by conscious feelings of being left out or not having what everyone else has. Other influences come from the people we interact with. Whatever their source, it serves to makes us feel like we have an incurable void only cured when we seek and devour the materialistic choices and treasures it is suggested we must have.

Characteristically, in these situations our urges are mental rather than bodily. Truly deconstructed such urges are really no more than a short-term fix of endorphins which don't negate the true cause of unhappiness.

As we edge further along the expectation line we find ourselves aspiring to stuff we can't have nor need and feel weak if we can't complete the task at hand in order to achieve them financially or physically. When we cannot complete the set task at hand in order to reach our expectation whether that be financially, mentally or physically we inevitably leave behind unresolved issues namely an uncompleted task. Where is the completion date? Is it days, weeks, years or decades ahead? Now the light at the end of the tunnel slowly extinguishes and is replaced by the darkness of unhappiness.

Often society intimates that the haves will always outdo the have-nots. That identity is reflected through the pot of gold or status quo within a social or work perspective. It is now highlighted by 21st century advertising techniques namely direct marketing whereby you 'suddenly' receive emails and advertising targeting those websites containing various products you may have looked at. As a result, our own sense of uniqueness can quickly be lost to a populace of likeminded and unimportant values and opinions.

Realistically we all live in part like this with our settings catered towards appeasing family, friends or our self. Often the very thing that aimed to unite the population in the search for acceptance, status quo and happiness does the opposite that is it deconstructs who we really are. What follows are enforcing excessive often pointless demands and requests on our time, money and personality whilst slowly detracting from who we truly are.

One has to focus on things that make happiness enjoyable. There must be a vow to learn and uphold the real you, to 'go to' a place in your life where you are safe and at terms with your values, opinions and morals keeping in mind that these will always be changing and adapting to the situations at foot moreover the times. And that always involves a chief ingredient of happiness - choice. Happiness is made difficult by a decision to choose one thing, person, or course of action in preference to others.[22].

Occasionally people may plan to hurt us and often there is no plan for unforeseen events however for the foreseen events the first step in the rest of our journey comes from choice.

Choice can often be muddied by differing opinion, social interaction, wisdom and maturity. People sometimes are smarter. Some foster false belief or negativity whilst some are forbidding with their thinking and acts. Sometimes we have no control over the choices we are presented with. For example, being an unwilling bystander at a robbery at the general store, watching a dog get hit by a car, seeing the devastation of an earthquake upon villages cannot be rectified by choice or positive thinking.

Even if one makes a concerted effort to always make the right choices one still has no control over the choices that other people make and this is one of the ingredients missing from the RECIPE of happiness. Occasionally, these obstacles in our happiness appear overwhelming. This is difficult. Difficult challenges don't have to be unachievable challenges. It is just a matter of adjusting your expectations.

Think you are alone?

The following list represents 7 people who have managed to remove the roadblock in their happiness, adjusted expectations, made choices and 'got' happy:

7. Derek Rabelo
'You have to believe in yourself. Go chase your dreams and you can do it if you want.'

So were some of the prophetic words of Derek Rabelo. Derek loves the feeling of salt water splashing his face and the rough and tumble of waves punishing and then caressing his body. Surfing is his passion and he shares the same waves that the world's elite ride upon every day. Derek as a professional surfer gets pounded in a tube and the surf often throws him around like rag doll in a playful dog's mouth yet he returns to the next set of waves to test his skill and precision.

Yet there is one thing that sets Derek aside from most of his competitors. Derek is blind. He was born with glaucoma yet he never considered his blindness a barrier to the ocean. His father presented him with surfboard on his 17th birthday and from that day he felt empowered by nature. Happiness invited him into its world.

Now he surfs the world toughest breaks, competing against others and himself no doubt struggling at times like we all do with what seem like insurmountable setbacks but are only challenges, 'Everybody feels frustrated sometimes. I never stopped to listen to the things that will not help me.' Along the way he considered the sea, 'Like energy and blessings and happiness. The best feeling in the world.'

6. Helen Keller
'The entire world is full of suffering. It is also full of overcoming.' - Helen Keller.

Helen Keller (June 27, 1880 – June 1, 1968) was an American author, political activist, and lecturer. She was the first deaf and blind person to earn a Bachelor of Arts degree (from Radcliffe College.) This was in 1904. Two years prior, in 1902, Helen Keller became the first person who was deaf and blind to write her autobiography, The Story of My Happiness.

Going on to become a prolific author, Keller was well-travelled and outspoken in her convictions. A member of the socialist party of America and the Industrial Workers of the World, she campaigned for women's suffrage, labour rights, socialism, and the common good.

"What we once enjoyed and deeply loved we can never lose, for all that we love deeply becomes a part of us."

5. Christopher Reeve, actor
'So many of our dreams at first seem impossible, then they seem improbable, and then, when we summon the will, they soon become inevitable.' Christopher Reeve,

Christopher Reeve achieved most of his fame for his portrayal of Superman - the man that was invincible and a national hero for his pretend world. In the real world Christopher Reeve was a champion in another way. He rose against the odds and challenged himself in a totally courageous way to make himself happy. Why?

After being thrown from a horse in 1995, the actor shattered his spine and was paralysed from the neck down. He was now a quadriplegic-unable to move from the neck down. The initial thoughts of suicide ran through his mind but even though he was severely disabled and worked with aid of a ventilator he revisited his ailment and challenged it.

He championed the cause of rehabilitation for severely spine-disabled people and encouraged research into spinal repair. Christopher Reeve was Voted Person of the Year in TIME magazine and his legacy the 'Christopher Reeves Spinal Foundation' still carries on his good work after his death in 2004.

'A Hero is an ordinary individual who finds the strength to persevere and endure in spite of overwhelming obstacles.' Christopher Reeve,

4. Kurt Fearnley

Kurt is an Australian who was born with a disorder called sacral agenesis which simply means he is missing certain parts of his lower spine and all of his sacrum.

At the time of birth, doctors did not believe he would live longer than a week.

But this didn't stop him. At school he took part in all sports including athletics and rugby league. He took up wheel chair racing at age 14 to train and post school completed a bachelor of human movement.

He participated in the Paralympic games in 2000, 2004, 2008, 2012 and 2016 collecting many medals along the way.

Yet in In November 2009 Fearnley at 41.4 metres in height and weighing just 50 kilograms was to face an even bigger challenge; he crawled the Kokoda trail in Papua New Guinea; famed World War 2 trail some 96 kilometres long defined by undulating, moral testing and body breaking terrain.

When asked why he chose to trek across such perilous terrain Fearnley responded with a candid statement which perhaps reflected his respect for life as whole -

'To keep it nice and simple I believed that I was strong enough to, I wanted to, and the 'why nots' just didn't add up.'

3. Ludwig van Beethoven, composer

'What you are, you are by accident of birth; what I am, I am by myself. There are and will be a thousand princes; there is only one Beethoven.'

To construct a symphony from scratch would be a monumental task for any aspiring or well-grounded artist. To be able to do so without being able to hear any of it would be almost impossible. 'Almost' because it was achieved by one Ludwig van Beethoven.

At the age of 26, armed with the strongest of strong mindset, Beethoven altered the course of musical history, even after he began to lose his hearing. Each year after he became progressively worse in deafness yet for the next 20 years he would compose some of his most influential pieces. One of those pieces included his phenomenal piece de resistance '9th Symphony' under a spectrum of a major hearing impediment - deafness.

'Off with you! You're a happy fellow, for you'll give happiness and joy to many other people. There is nothing better or greater than that!' Ludwig van Beethoven.

2. Oprah Winfrey, TV personality

'I am a woman in process. I'm just trying like everybody else. I try to take every conflict, every experience, and learn from it. Happiness is never dull.' Oprah Winfrey

Oprah Gail Winfrey was born to a teenage single mother, underprivileged and penniless, in rural Mississippi. She was often dressed in used potato sacks from her early years. Winfrey has stated she was molested by her cousin, uncle, and a family friend, starting when she was nine years old.

At 13, after suffering years of abuse, Winfrey ran away from home. In her early teens (aged 14) she gave birth to a son who died in infancy. And what was her mindset?

She adopted the desire to work forward in happiness. She was motivated to work in media and nurtured her own career through study and experience. She left no stone unturned in order to improve her happiness in any way she could.

Today, Oprah is one of the most influential women in the world; an influential giver of time, money, encouragement and patience.

'Be thankful for what you have; you'll end up having more. If you concentrate on what you don't have, you will never, ever have enough.' Oprah Winfrey

1. Mother Teresa

Mother Teresa founded the missionaries of Charity, which in 2012 is active in 133 countries. They run hospices and homes for people with HIV/AIDS, leprosy and tuberculosis; soup kitchens; dispensaries and mobile clinics; children's and family counselling programmes; orphanages; and schools.

She was born Agnes Gonxha Bojaxhiu on August 26, 1910. Her father, who was involved in Albanian politics, died in 1919 when she was eight years old. She chose a happiness of happiness derived from helping others and over a period of time she changed the face and dynamics of care for the poor.

During her long life of helping the less fortunate she herself faced many obstacles:
...A heart attack in Rome in 1983, while visiting Pope John Paul 11

...Suffered a second attack in 1989, she received a pacemaker

...In 1991, after a battle with pneumonia while in Mexico, she suffered further heart problems

...In April 1996, Mother Teresa fell and broke her clavicle (collarbone). In August of the same year she suffered from malaria and failure of the left heart ventricle. She died a short time later.

In her time, she penned an ode to life and in particular the beauty that rests within each and every breath:

'Happiness is an opportunity, benefit from it. Happiness is beauty, admire it.
Happiness is a dream, realize it. Happiness is a challenge, meet it.
Happiness is a duty, complete it. Happiness is a game, play it.
Happiness is a promise, fulfil it. Happiness is sorrow, overcome it.
Happiness is a song, sing it. Happiness is a struggle, accept it.
Happiness is a tragedy, confront it. Happiness is an adventure, dare it.
Happiness is luck, make it. Happiness is too precious, do not destroy it.
Happiness is happiness, fight for it.'
- Mother Teresa

People have had many devastating things happen to them and to the people they love but that does not mean there are no exciting things that will greet people in the future. That is there are lots of things to look forward to doing and seeing – to you and your friends/family.

Let`s take some encouragement:

I. Be glad of happiness because it gives one the chance to utilise your senses; to love work, play, listen, sing, read, feel and to look at everything around you.

ii. The age-old quotation 'this too shall pass.' sums up most frustrating situations especially if one constructs ways to address the 'This'. A festering sore will not heal with wishful thinking. It needs an approach - treatment. Plan your approach and ask for constructive criticism then under judgement carry it forward.

THE SECRET RECIPE TO FEELING GREAT INSTANTLY!

6. Awareness

There is no doubt the mind plays a huge part in determining outcomes. As we touched upon prior the mindset has the utmost importance; in sport, relationships, work and culture. A derivative of mind games involves both Positivity and Awareness.

Positivity benefits the guardians of our body the immune system helping people cope with life's obstacles, unfortunate news and events which threaten to weaken our demeanour.

Awareness simply means conscious of life's' up s and downs - offering no excuses.

Both positivity and awareness influence building a stronger and henceforth happier you. People who are more positive and aware of their life have greater responses to life's setbacks and appreciate the things in life which underpin true joy. They approach from an understanding of what they have not what they don't thereby fuelling positivity and ensuring happiness. Often this results in giving to others and relating to the community on a constant basis. There is almost a loss of self-centredness and indulgence. Recent research indicates that positive people and those aware of their life and negative people or those always willing and needing the next big thing approach problems differently and vary greatly in their ability to cope successfully with adversity and privilege .

We have to work every day, sunrise to sunset, just to survive. However, we often think we face insurmountable challenges and maybe our lives seem difficult because we think we 'can`t do'. Socrates (469-399BC) sweet-talked his fellow countrymen to muse the realms of truth and justice, 'the unexamined life is not worth living.'

Socrates belied happiness is reachable by human determination, acquisition of coherent control over one's cravings and coordinating the varied highs and lows of your emotion. This in turn would lead to inner peace which any dent to the outer would not affect. This was somewhat against current thought at that time for most believed happiness was privy for those whom the gods deemed sovereign or holy. Consequently, in a nutshell Socrates preferred the moral life to an immoral one perhaps underpinned not by want or desire but by virtues; justice and love.

Sometimes, our desire is what makes happiness difficult. Paradoxically to Socrates' musings imagine if we lived in a world where no one had any desire and we all passively accepted our lives - there would be no research or advancement in technology, building, arts or health.

Happiness is simple but puzzlingly even in an active role it can come unstuck simply through embarking on too many tasks without adequate preparation, thought or involvement which in turn can quickly be set with complication. That is multi-tasking and without groundwork can lead to multi-stuff-ups. However, the desire to solve even the most intricate of problems is a gift not a burden for if this problem chose you it`s more than likely that it knew you could solve it.

We can all progress and be happy and this simply understands a few points of interest more neatly:
...Sometimes in our happiness we are subjected to events outside our control.
...Most of us don't go around inviting unwanted trials into our lives. Still, from time to time we do need to deal with them. What's important in these situations is not so much the event but how we respond to it. When we find ourselves in that situation, our awareness and positivity will definitely influence how we view the experience and in turn how we cope with it.
...However, it is important we have the necessary tools in place in order to make an assessment. By implementing these few skillsets, we can assess and work our way through any event.

7 Ways to refuse to be unhappy:

1. Remove your-self emotionally.
Most adverse and self-deflating events are usually met with adverse and self-deflating emotions. When one refuses to be involved, the situation is rendered neutral. Now rational thought is at the forefront of action instead of adrenaline charged irrationality.

2. Ask How and what?
How can I solve the problem at hand?
How will I ensure safety morals and understanding come into play?
What steps can I take to create a sensible and workable solution?
What steps will ensure people maintain their dignity and self-esteem?

3. Look for the lesson in it all.
What value is there in the challenge?
a. In front of you or
 B. Ahead of you.
What is it teaching me?

4. Seek guidance.
There are always smarter people then yourself. Seek and learn from their experience and knowledge.

5. Nothing lasts forever – 'This too shall pass.'
Note it's temporary.
The sun is always shining but sometimes it is hidden behind clouds.

6. Third man. Take the view of an innocent bystander, a third man, to any event thrust upon you. How would he or she see the event in which you find yourself and how would they use it to turn an adverse and self-deflating into a positive? Turn challenges into opportunities.

7. Don't take it personally. Sometimes it can feel like you are the 'chosen one' to face more than your fair share of challenges. Don`t encourage adverse and self-deflating thinking. Moreover the 'Why me?' syndrome should be placed in the nearest dumpster. If Helen Keller to Mother Teresa didn`t entertain the 'Why me?' syndrome then probably it`s fair to say you shouldn`t either.

How to Become Happier

1. Give permission to be human: Accept emotions, even fright, despondency and worry serves some purpose to happiness. Rejecting them leads to denial and anger.

2. Go quietly amongst the racket and rush of life.

3. Find meaning and pleasure: Engage in goals we want to achieve versus what we feel obliged to do, spend two hours per week with our hobbies, spend time with our loved ones, etc.

4. Focus on the positive, on what works well for us, and be grateful. Write 5 things every day before you sleep that you are grateful for, even seemingly minuscule things like the smile of someone close, the sound of birds chirping, and so on.

5. Increase the effort you put into your relationships. Go on a date with your wife or your husband or spend more time speaking to your children.

6.Simplify: We need to do less. Pin point your concentration i.e. Focus on one thing at the time, eliminate multitasks and don't read complications into what feels humble.

7.Be aware of the mind-body connection: Exercise, practice mindfulness meditation, yoga, and breathing exercises. An experiment conducted on three groups of people (one exercising, one on medication, the last one on both) for four months showed that 38 % of the group on medication went back on depression, against 9 % in group who exercised (Lyubomirsky 1998).

8.Shun brash and violent people – they are distressing to the spirit.

9. Speak quietly, clearly and listen to others.

10.Call upon calm, silence, consideration and communication in the face of fear and trauma.

11.Take pride in your efforts and the achievements of others.

7. Heading towards the Happy Spot

The meaning of happiness is a metaphysical inquiry concerning the worth of happiness or survival overall. It can also be communicated in different forms, such as 'Where do we come from?', 'Who are we?', and 'Where are we going?' It has been the subject of much debate throughout the ages not sparing philosophical, scientific, and theological opinion. The answer springs from a background pertaining to education often underpinned by culture and ideology.

In recent times, the media has perpetuated the myth that happiness can be obtained through materialistic pleasure namely status, money, looks, fame and notoriety.

If we fall into this clumsy trap, we will be stuck in a world full of despair and spite which leads one down the resentment track.

Perhaps the easiest way to bag the happy spot is to keep things as simple as possible, whilst entertaining that most complicated matters need only to be looked at without selfish ulterior motives and the illogical, unreasonable and enemy within that seeks to champion it.

Theodore Geisel, or as you know him, Dr Seuss the famed author of the Cat in the hat books amidst others, once famously stated, 'Don't cry because it's over, smile because it's happened.' Whilst Ralph Waldo Emerson confided to a work colleague (and millions of others!),'For every minute you are angry you lose sixty seconds of happiness.'

True happiness can only be attained through true worth – of yourself, those around you and from that which makes you a better person. But keep in mind every now and then our moral compass is bound to wobble. With that in mind and in order to invite happy let us embrace the following:

Hints for Happiness

- Savour happiness

'Happiness is free. Freedom has no price. Perhaps it should.'

Take the time to smell, feel, touch and listen to the beauty around. Mother Nature is always there and all it takes is a little time each day.

In the past few decades the importance of Mother Nature and the contact with the natural world for human health, well-being and functioning has been amply documented by research.

A 2009 study by Kaplan et al showed that taking a walk in a park has paybacks for both attention and memory: after spending 60 minutes in nature both increased by 20 per cent. The results show that this effect does not occur for those who took a walk in an urban area.

The researchers found that even when participants observed images, of natural environments and urban environments, those observing the natural ones did better on the attention and memory tests. The authors suggested that being outside in the natural surroundings fulfils straightforward needs and produces parallel results to meditating.1

Therefore, consider this:
a. Mother Nature helps to negate the stress and strain of everyday happiness.
b. Mother Nature encourages us to reason with our problems and place them in perspective i.e. a warrant list. Does this problem warrant consideration and if so without worry?
c. Mother Nature is a collage of beauty and it affectively puts in balance our appreciation of true beauty.
d. Mother Nature is an environment that encourages peace, tranquillity and happiness and it`s free!
All of this helps to promote free, clear and concise thinking strengthened by the sight, smell, touch and sound of Mother Nature.

The following gives a few specific examples of research on the benefits of contact with the natural world:
A study by Russell and Mehrabian in 1976 verified that screening people visions of pleasing natural scenes promoted positive health awareness thereby quelling the desire to participate in unhealthy behaviours such as drugs, including smoking, and alcohol.

The benefit of even limited contact with nature does not only limit itself to the physical component of health but also encompasses the mental state as well. This is achieved mainly through the reduction of stress and worry. And so, the cycle continues for now mental serenity feeds-back to the physical since reducing stress effects the cardiovascular system.

A 2007 research project carried out by the University of Essex even showed that a walk in the country could counteract depression. *

2. Never compare yourself
Never compare yourself to others for there will always be person greater or lesser then you. Your own achievements, however humble, are important as any.

Throw away the tabloids, the cosmetically enhanced celebrity telling you beauty lies in this or that product. Ignore the trumpeting of the business leaders who urge you to own it all or the so-called investment gurus who want you to be rich. Play deaf ears with those who tell and encourage you to aspire to the 'greater' gain of cars, bicycles, houses and playthings.

When you seek to compare yourself to other people and their happiness styles, it is quite common to draw the conclusion that you lack something, and you become overwhelmed with dissatisfaction. However, to do this raises many queries:

a. You have no true idea how the other half lives. It is not uncommon for the so called glamorous happiness to be buttressed by debt, despondency, resentment and bewilderment

b. You are effectively rating your happiness on a scale and no empirical value can do justice for laughter, empathy, comfort and appreciation. The way forward is always littered with those who believe they are 'above' or 'beyond' others – those looking aimlessly for bragging rights and isolated in despondency.

c. Comparisons are always unbalanced. So, it may mean we view comparison as meaning the worst of this versus the best of that and the only thing that achieves is narcissism – not the noblest of badges.

d. Comparisons rob your-self of time. When we are busy comparing we are not doing.

e. The world is never a level playing field. Materialistically there are always imbalances as there are with knowledge, literature, oratory, sporting and musical talent. So, it is an endless road in seeking comparison and a road littered with creating self-indulgence, vanity and self-centredness

"Comparison is the thief of joy" - Theodore Roosevelt

3. Love yourself - wants and needs

Love yourself – create time, space and needs for you. Wants are just that 'wants'. Instead of aiming for the want of materialistic pleasures purposefully seek out the path to a happier you from those 'needs' – good friends, loving family and good people.

Embrace true values. They media seem to overflow the T.V, radio, internet, glossy magazine and cinema with images of the rich, and beautiful.
They uphold this image constantly and a feeling of inadequacy evolves. It serves to create chinks in our armour. But love, truth, honour, respect and empathy are values to

uphold the happy and enamour our body with a shield of steel. It was Kaint who said, 'We are not rich by what we possess but by what we can do without.'

'When you can look in the mirror and smile only then can your smile be felt by others.'

4. Be yourself

Be self-effacing and that simply means: Modest, unassuming, and unpretentious. People who announce their 'greatness' or who are the proverbial 'I am King' are usually those who are the weakest link in times when a steely resolve is needed.

There is no victory in seeking the buried treasure of materialistic pleasure. Be enamoured with the strength of knowledge instead of the weakness of dollars. Keep in mind no one can find it hard to be happy if they don`t pay the electricity bill so making ends meet is still important but to be overcome by the lure of a dollar bill can lure unhappiness and promote egotism, conceit and narcissism.

'To be yourself in a world that is constantly trying to make you something else is the greatest accomplishment.' - Ralph Emerson.

5. Strengthen your family ties

George Burns once commented about happiness, 'Happiness is having a large, loving caring close-knit family in another city.'

Laughable at first but on second consideration, in these constantly changing times where we constantly procrastinate and strive for some sort of immortality, the close support network of family can never be underestimated. Moreover, those who share their life with others intent on forgiving and giving more, who smile, listen, accept and understand, create their own family of sorts. As such it doesn't have to be immediate but also can be formed amongst friends. The benefits are enormous; be willing to invite the trials and challenges into life; encourage self- content the workhorse of all happiness; build self-esteem; create feedback and unconditional support and perhaps most of all love.

6. 'Live your life through someone else's eyes.'

The hardest thing to do even imagine is to walk in someone else's shoes. Yet perhaps to achieve real happiness I believe the change we must navigate and accept is that which

admits the ebbs and flows of life of the next person. When we ALL strip life down to its basics we appreciate that we all experience angst and regret but experience much more love and friendship.

The balance is everything and the equilibrium we all must look toward is the balance of what is right, wrong, destructive, constructive, understanding and denial. Only from helping others realize and recognize this do we experience happiness within.

References:

Arbor, A, 2008, 'Going outside- even in the cold-improves memory, attention, University of Michigan News Service.

Berman, M. G., Jonides, J & Kaplan, S., 2008, 'The Cognitive Benefits of Interacting With Nature', Psychological Science, 19(12), 1207-1212.

Burns, G. W, 2005, 'Naturally happy, naturally healthy: the role of the natural environment in well-being' in Huppert, F. A., Baylis, N., & Keverne, B, 2005, The Science of Well-being, Oxford University Press.

Kaplan, S., 1995, 'The Restorative Benefits of Nature: Towards An Integrative Framework.', Journal of Environmental Psychology, 15, 169-182.

Mitchell, R., & Popham, F., 2008, 'Effect of exposure to natural environment on health inequalities: an observational population study', 272(9650), 1655-1660.

University of Sheffield 2007 Media Centre news release, 'There's much more to a walk in the park'.

8. A Great Person
...GUARANTEED

A Great Person seeks no approval or judgement. He or she seeks no adulation or ego fill. There is no need to fill the trophy cabinet. But that doesn`t mean one lowers expectations or standards in due measure. Instead the happy person always tests their own limits and grows from within.

Be who you can be and that is done by striving to your ability in everything. But don`t set unrealistic expectations. This is not a competition. It is your happiness. Strive to be enlightened.

Happiness with Meaning
Viktor Frankl wrote in *man's search for meaning* that 'Everything can be taken from a man but one thing...the last of the human freedoms – to choose one's attitude in any given set of circumstances, to choose one's own way.'

Whether one is a sportsman, parliamentarian, electrician, musician, gardener, father, or student we are all founded by intention, response and commitment. * We have a thought to achieve and we respond then commit to it. That is happiness with meaning. To want happiness to create your meaning is totally wrong...your meaning creates your happiness.

Case study
Roma was always on the receiving end. Receiving gifts, help, and advice and going about her daily life always thankful for small mercies and the love she got every day. She was also on the receiving end of war torn Italy, the depression and the countless years of war. A widower she lived her life the way she wanted others to live.

86-year-old Roma was constantly aware of the help from her community and always gave back. She put down her happiness and to her meaning. She found a way to appreciate others she offered her words of wisdom in preparing food and even showed her skills to those who couldn't bake or make ends meet on a small budget. She consistently showed others that giving thanks for the good things in her life made her appreciative of love and kindness. She was openly thankful for the contribution of others and acknowledged that openly. She would often call upon someone with a word, card or a simple gift. She called it gratitude and it was just a part of what makes her happy.

It is never too late to simply give thanks. Roma would often say strive to be the best possible versions of yourself—not only for your own self, but for the benefit and contribution you can offer to others.

Work hard to take care of yourself physically and emotionally and show others how it can be done by just being you.

Albert Einstein famously uttered 'Only happiness lived for others are happiness worthwhile.' Perhaps he was alluding to Roma yet when we truly think about giving we can define some important facts:

- Giving leads to understanding what's happening in someone's happiness.

b. Giving makes us feel happy. A 2008 study by Harvard Business School professor Michael Norton and colleagues found that giving money to someone else lifted participants' happiness more that spending it on themselves

In a 2006 study, Jorge Moll and colleagues at the National Institute of Health found that when people give to charities, it switched on the brain pleasure, social attachment and hope centres - like telephone switchboard lighting up - encouraging a release of a slightly euphoric high – possibly the endorphin (feel good) hormone in play.

c.Giving is good for our health. A wide range of research has linked different forms of generosity to better health. Stephanie Brown of the University of Michigan in 2003 and her colleagues found those who gave as such had a lower risk of dying (possibly as a result of decreased stress) over a five-year period than those who didn't.

d. Giving promotes cooperation and social connection. When you give, you're more likely to get back: Several studies, by sociologists Simpson and Willer, have suggested that giving is rewarded by others along the way.

Cooperation strengthens our ties to others—and research has shown that having positive social interactions encourages a healthy mental and physical state.

e. Giving evokes gratitude. Whether you're on the giving or receiving end of a gift, it can be a way of expressing gratitude or instilling gratitude in the recipient.

A recent study led by Nathaniel Lambert at Florida State University established that conveying gratitude to a friend or partner fortifies a connection to that person. Moreover, what the connection underpins is a growing relationship and silently conveys morals, boundaries and values

f. Giving is contagious. A study published in the Proceedings of the National Academy of Science by Fowler and Christakis, shows that when one person behaves generously, it inspires a domino effect. The generosity is now passed on later, toward different people – '…each person in a network can influence dozens or even hundreds of people, some of whom he or she does not know and has not met.'

g. Giving has also been linked to the release of oxytocin, a hormone (also released during sex) that induces feelings of warmth, euphoria, and connection to others. In laboratory studies, Paul Zak, at Claremont Graduate University, has found that a dose of oxytocin will cause people to give more generously and to feel more empathy towards others unfortunately it only lasted for two hours…still. Giving makes you feel good and it may come in many forms: Money, goods and services (old and new), skills, expertise, random acts of kindness, time and patience.

Case study
Neil was a welfare recipient for over the last twenty years from 1993 to 2013.
He managed to wean himself from his psychological profile of being poor and low in esteem mainly by seeing then accepting himself for who he was not through the eyes or acceptance of others. He was one person who also shaped the way I learned to think. You see many people feel the need to be completely approved of yet being clearly admired by people is nigh impossible and implausible. There will be many people in your life that you just don't and won't gel with. Often the reasons are unknown yet due to the simple nature of varying views, opinions, cultures and religious plays they may stick out like an open car door.

Often it is their view of you which plays an important role in defining who they are as people. If there is no apparent reason then it stands to question whether there are other motives at play (e.g., spite, envy, hurtful or bigoted attitudes, social ineptitude etc.) Often the waters are muddied in reflection.
What is clear, however, is that the waters only become murkier and almost quick sand like when we try to foster public approval. Quite simply it is a recipe for unhappiness.

Case study:
Gerard thought he had to meet others expectation of him from an early age at school and through university. What this ensured for him was a journey through medication addiction both prescribed and illicit. His journey met with obstacle after obstacle, yet it was only when he had an epiphany (as he called it) in late 2012 whilst watching a leading rock band perform on stage that his views or expectations changed.

He listened in intermission as the patrons in one corner complained of poor performance whilst those in the other corner were enraptured. He realised no matter how hard the rock band tried and no matter what they would say, sing or do, there were inevitably going to be some people who just didn't like them or their performance.

He soon realised personally that trying to gain people's approval will require that he distort, twist and convolute himself into something that wasn't him and often we do this by getting ourselves into atypical group situations, socially, culturally even with work acquaintances which forfeits our own genuineness in the passage defined by unrealistic expectation of ourselves in trying to do things through another's eyes.

True acceptance, doesn't seek or need approval and/or affection from others.
Feeling this was one of the chief reasons of his unhappiness he sought other rewards for happiness and managed to hold a job for the first time in some 2 years on a constant basis.

Case study
Billy aged 36 had everything and nowhere to put it. A merchant banker he was not short of what many describe as the treasure chest of happiness; money, materials and mystery yet there was always the feeling he needed to be better than the next person.

As a boss if he was better than his workforce them he was happier than them. This was the pecking order of authority and control; therefore, he didn't appreciate the next person. Years of this set up a situation where Billy only had the company of one, himself, at lunch and down time, and although seeming contented with his materialistic life the company of one soon made for a strange and shallow bedfellow.

Soon the self- appraisal began and quickly, like many of the stints in abuse, beggared the introduction and nurturing of: Promiscuity, indulgence in drugs and alcohol and the crushing impact of reflection. After a brief stint in rehab he realised that in order to be happy he had to readjust his definition of happiness and that started with appreciating others.

His goal was simple in the extreme: Try to cultivate and nourish a few genuine, intimate relationships. This way he could free himself of the toxic tendency to favour fair weather acquaintances.
This was a somewhat simple task in its extreme done by focusing instead on a much smaller amount of real, authentic friends who, it was hoped, would genuinely yet slowly and politely offer ways to improve himself.

Case study

Noelene l had been a welfare recipient for 40 years. This was an unwritten clause in her life passed down from generation to generation; even her daughter was on welfare just 'because I can'.

It was only the last 6 years that Noelene finally discovered the value of giving. Noelene was always taking but hardly giving. This all changed when someone close to her was dying and Noelene offered not only companionship but help around the home and in daily tasks; she was often called upon to go shopping and provide showering for her friend.

It was this component of happiness – giving – that lead to aged care work and which encouraged a similar path for her daughter.

Sure, some people do need welfare, and some don't. If you feel that you can give something back to the community don't hesitate.

Case study

Ferus found his life felt depleted of enjoyment. He couldn't savour any delights and struggled for momentum in any form of happiness. He soon just through some quite introspection discovered what was subtracting from his life, 'looking forward to doing meaningful things.'

Often, the meaningful things are humble pleasures of life. This may simply be: A walk, a hot bath, running an errand for someone; mowing some's lawn for instance, listening to enjoyable music. For many of us planning grander things like taking a vacation, buying yourself a gift, a romantic interlude can be a source of great, enthusiastic anticipation, as well but almost always the simple pleasures are best, more meaningful and longer lasting in satisfaction and I simply call that 'devoting time.'

Case study
Julia

Julia lived a life of intense pressure. A child prodigy she was constantly ahead of where she was supposed to be and for a 4-year-old doing piano recitals and as an 8-year-old discovering she had the talents of an 18-year-old the journey became somewhat foggy in her study and social detail.

 She got lost through poor guidance and sign posts with no real mentor outside of pushy parents who thought they were doing what was best for their kid. She struggled mostly with the alienation of not being able to be around 8-year old's and do other 8-year-old things; comic book reading, music, play games, mingling, tell stories and giggle too much. Her life was serious, and she knew it until one day some 6 years later as adolescence overwhelmed her she wondered why she didn't attract any true friends and it dawned on her that all this seriousness never really allowed her to let her smile out.

You know one main ingredient in happiness is just to smile, sounds trivial, doesn't it? But as Julia was soon to find out smiling does something scientifically proven; it stimulates the production of endorphins.

When our brains feel happy, endorphins are manufactured, and nerves fire up along their transport network; brain to your facial muscles and a smile is produced. And when you really think about it a second smile is never too far off. The cycle of happiness is underway. Research indicates when our smiling muscles turn on the body releases the feel-good hormone, endorphins, which encourage us to feel happy and this encourages the mind and body to feel energised, uplifts the spirit and there is an addiction in place prompting us to do it all again; to smile again. It is simply a positive action and reaction.

A Swedish study found that seeing people smile stimulates our own neurones to trigger a smile. Furthermore, smiling also brings health benefits, like reducing worry, as well as lowering your blood pressure and heart rate.

Charles Darwin first posed the idea that emotional responses influence our feelings in 1872. 'The free expression by outward signs of an emotion intensifies it,' he wrote.
One study at the University of Cardiff in Wales found that people whose ability to frown is 'rejected' by injections of Botox are reportedly happier, on middling, than people who can frown. 'It would appear that the way we feel emotions isn't just restricted to our brain.'

There are parts of our bodies that help and reinforce our feelings - so suggested Michael Lewis, who co-wrote the study. '...it feeds back to the body.'
The concept works the opposite way, too—enhancing emotions rather than suppressing them. People who frown during an unpleasant procedure report feeling more pain than those who do not, according to a study published in May 2008 in the Journal of Pain. 'It's possible that people may feel less pain if they're unable to express it,' it says.

But we have all heard that it is bad to repress our feelings—so what happens if a person intentionally suppresses his or her adverse and self-deflating emotions on an ongoing basis? What if we continue to bottle our angst, dismay or dissatisfaction?

Work by psychologist Judith Grob, of the University of Groningen in the Netherlands suggests that this stifled negativity may 'leak' into other realms of a person's happiness.

In fact, a study of those who repressed their emotion and those in the control group had notable outcomes: Those with repressed emotion virtually fostered pessimism as evident through memory tasks and missing letter tasks. For instance, they completed 'gr_ss' as 'gross' rather than 'grass,' as compared with the control group. 'People who tend to do this regularly might start to see the world in a more adverse and self- deflating light,' Grob says.

Even facial and body gestures play a role – 'When the face doesn't aid in expressing the emotion, the emotion seeks other channels to express itself through.' Grob added.

So, a simple smile changed the way Julia looked at almost everything and it paid big dividends combing her skillsets with a list of friends her own age and older with who she spent many happy fun times together both at work and at socially.

Case study
Doug 66
Einstein famously championed, 'A person starts to live when he can live outside himself.'

Doug was busy being himself. The life of the party the one who could talk under water, whose opinion was the right one, who proverbially felt like and acted like the sun shone from one part of his anatomy. We have all met them. Yet when it came to quality one on one time and family time he was both clueless and a mess. He had developed fractured relationships with his past 3 wives and families and even friends gave him the short shift.

Often, we don't realise we are morphing into a Doug when the 'I am' man comes out in us; 'I do this, I do that, I did this, I believe that, I want this, I am owed that.'

Families and friends are but passing acquaintances who soon become peeved and offer an excuse or ten not are in your company. Yet taking time to read some self- help books (after a Christmas party left him drinking with his shadow) he soon instigated some homework and changed his ways. Doug made time to reflect on why he felt 'incomplete'.

Family and friends are invaluable. They are the greatest source of contact who offers help, empathy and companionship in times of despair and unhappiness.

Sometimes we feel like our happiness isn't exciting because we're only doing the work that we need to do in order to get by. Take time to do work for someone else and having mastered that work take on a new hobby or maybe learn something different like a new language with someone. Invite warm companionship and not only will one`s time be spent doing something productive, but you'll have a sense of satisfaction when you make progress on both accounts.

The results are impressive: Now we can set the accomplished task in stone i.e. set within the framework of our brain, so it is easier to recall.

There is nothing quite like the companionship, laughter and guidance that family and friends portray in times of learning new tasks. Happiness does not have to impress anyone. And just like Doug learned there is value in people outside oneself and by taking interest, listening and communicating the fractured relationship soon heals, love becomes unconditional and hope arises for a better and happier you.

There is no doubting the number of hurdles we have to jump in order to remain on a peaceful happy passage in life. Despite the fact human error and unforeseen circumstances chip away at our happiness and sometimes with great immediate consequence there are many ingredients which help make the recipe for happiness fulfilling in its entirety. There are also many which spoil the recipe. Throw them out and let the happiness rise!

* Michael Father Senior - 'EVER STATE' in 'How to Survive the Death of a Loved One', Amazon.

9. Getting the best out of a bad situation

Happiness is an emotional and physical feeling of comfort that incorporates living with an understanding of consequence and deep fulfilment. Feeling great usurps this on a constant basis!

Studies reveal that happiness is not some leap frog from one treasure chest to another in the form of short term adrenalin rushes or endorphin fix as we chase pleasures instantly. Rather Research shows that happiness characteristically comprises intervals of considerable discomfort. Many would assign the word negativity to this word 'discomfort'.

Sure, finances contribute to happiness but not as much as the magazine scribes and advertising agencies would have you believe. Money buys lack of restrictions from worry about the basics in life—where we live, what we eat and what we wear. But truly we are made of genetic variances, subjected to fluctuating circumstances, inherit and condition our feelings, achieve, choose our marital status, embrace social relationships and nurture our own communal input according to how we want and when we want to influence happiness at any time.

Scientists approximate that considerable happiness lies within our perception and understanding of what matters most in life. They suggest indulging in small pleasures self-pampering, removing one's self from the comfort lounge to challenge, creating realistic goals, keeping up friendships, and realising ones importance without seeking admiration are all engagements that encourage happiness.

But there are many detractors from happiness that one must be aware of. The detractors are important because they signify how happy you are and whether you have the ability to swing them around in your favour. More noteworthy is that these detractors are real and there is no dodging them. Hiding from them erodes happiness whilst meeting them head on helps to foster happiness. So, you see the detractors can easily become the champion of your happiness!

Such detractors are the adverse and self-deflating emotions we feel at various times; some more than others. Considered nuisance value and demeaning these emotions are in fact are a first aid pack. They emotionally save us from ourselves. Calls of 'I'm an idiot' or 'why did I stuff that up?', or 'I failed that task' reeks of emotional attachment, quite simply it is us not completing a task to our expectation or desire. It is like an alarm bell sounding in this case to remind us to adjust what we're undertaking and readjust our thoughts and actions. These adverse or self-deflating emotions are required for good mood.

However, emotions that continue to generate unpleasant feelings for instance resentment, spite, defeat, sorrow, grief, blame and shame are often not verbalised but often stifled and /or medically numbed and we ridicule our self for their 'uprising' whilst berating out loud for the happiness eroded in us.

Whilst this is manifesting beneath our surface a change occurs in inspiration, functioning, consideration, awareness, principles, and actions ranging from: Worrying, snickering, payback, confidence, and memory regression. Whilst it seems that each change looks to take us down a peg or two in fact it is teaching us to move onwards in our journey whether it is about to concoct unwanted advice, intrusion or exclusion.

Whatever way you look at it these adverse emotions all in some way help us work through the human experience suggesting methods of repair, intervention, prevention and perhaps conclusion to some if not most of life's frailties, indiscretions and problems.

Quite clearly to be imbued by the true meaning of life we need to accept and endure its challenges as well as the attached emotions good and not so good. It is only then when we know how to accept and deal with these emotions that we can truly invite happiness into not only our life but others: Resentment, fright and worry.

Resentment
Resentment and the attached fury can feel like a volcano within erupting for everyone to see through built up blasts of energy, almost always igniting those emotions we often feel disappointed with our selves post circumstance. Your heart pumps furiously, the perspiration gathers like a potential flood, your blood boils, you create the road of revenge seeking what is right according to your values and morals and how you manage to communicate it – often rapidly and haphazardly.

These emotions have the ability to override even the calm in all of us depending of course on the circumstances. Further still if you can see the repercussion of something and someone echoes their sentiments resentment arises.

However, the attached emotion to resentment serves something good - it opens up emotions and lets them out. No stifling or harbouring thoughts or ill worlds or god forbid actions.
The extent to which you deliver such thoughts words and actions need to be reined in otherwise an eye for an eye never solved anything. Controlled rational discussion does.

Of course, this varies with cultural differences and personalised choices, but external release is not such a bad thing. It perhaps promotes closure to matters of interest and importance bringing them forward faster and with more passion.

And resentment does not simply benefit the individual. It also highlights equality, champion human rights and uphold values. For those in relationships venting and arguing can be away of therapeutically clearing grievances and creating clarity for the past, present and future.

Adverse and self- deflating experience can be the impetus to reassessing your qualifications and capabilities with job choices making sure you don't aim too high or too low.

So, you see defeat, sorrow, grief, blame and shame not to mention self-consciousness always impact on our happiness but they can fuel it as well. Even though you may feel bad after getting retrenched or sacked from a team it is not the same emotion attached to say making such a mistake like falling off a bike for no reason.

The discomfort of, defeat, sorrow, grief, blame and shame invite retrospection as well as introspection to encourage a better you however the process can be somewhat intimidating. The 'beauty' of them is that they invite ownership of mistakes and concurrent to the above emotions leads to making good. This making good may take the form of mending what you damaged, listening and cooperation or by reorganising thoughts and words, opinions and values and giving assistance to others.

Involuntarily, happiness is predisposed by a pecking order of sorts, I have this they don't. I am above them in my mind and apparently in the social status quo. Whilst nothing is further from the truth this impression even though fleeting can ignite a stronger work ethic to achieve more and be more productive. The worry and for some embarrassment of being less than others re material worth gets neatly confined within a basketful of shame, blame and jealousy whilst paradoxically helping to reduce or reverse inferiority, to feather one's own nest. That in itself can lead to more confidence and self -worth, clearer values and views.

However, happiness will still be underpinned by a context of sense and morals and no amount of one upmanship will ever lead to happiness on a longer level it may even breed dissatisfaction and disenchantment if one expects to achieve a certain spot in the pecking order and doesn't. Never the less the ignition switch to be better at what you do encourages a better mood and that is one ingredient of the recipe of happiness.

Yet it doesn't mean we should yell abuse or become jealous to achieve happiness as a whole. Far from it. What it does do is jolts us with a dose of reality. For all the running training we may do we may never ever eclipse Usain Bolt's long-standing track sprint records. Owning up to reality is important. Bolt is a better runner and perhaps you would appreciate with your own training what it took for him to be successful.

Liken that to work, social and intimate relationships and what first appeared as the sins of life now appear as treasures.

Fright and Worry

Fright aids our body to prepare for battle. It encompasses the surge of adrenalin to fight or flee. It challenges us to decide between risk and reward or risk and danger or no risk.

Think about it. Without fright, we become naïve danger seekers. Even that aside there will be many moments as we passage through life there when our judgement becomes clouded either through maturity (pre-teenage and teenage years), intoxication (any age past 13) and ill health (all ages). And those danger seeking naïve moments can lead to anything from unprotected sex to economic collapse. Sometimes the consequences aren't solid and we only sense on the full impact of our misdemeanour or unhappiness from the after effect.

But sooner or later we all are faced with a dose of reality and even intermittent worry about the direction of our life can cause us to change redirect our focus to where it is warranted, readjust values and opinions and uphold our true worth. So, a small dose of. worry can serve a remedial almost restorative purpose, helping us to reassess ourselves.

Yes, there is some element of strength in fright and worry just; not too much of it. Overdosing on it or if one struggles to confront the threat and seek remedy then blame, shame and worry may have bigger more destructive consequences.

10. The Crown of Greatness– Full of Patience, regret, dissatisfaction, despondency and other Happiness blockers?

Patience is a virtue
With patience you can control your thoughts. Control your thoughts before they control you. Patience is the most important of all the virtues, because without it you cannot see what unfolds and decide whether to accept or deny it. It is possible to stretch too far. We never really get the guardian angel sitting on our shoulder tapping away when we are about to go in the wrong moral direction offering some form of honourable guidance. In its simplest form if a view shaped a difficulty in your life then the same view won`t remove it.

Patience is vital in happiness and perhaps the one key sub ingredient which many people fail to utilise to its full capacity in order to achieve happiness is to listen.

The benefits of being an active patient listener are incalculable. They range from increased knowledge to more compassion. Patient Listening is a hallmark of happy people. It is a skill practiced by so few that to be able to do it well sets one apart from the pack.

Some of the benefits of patient listening include:
- One is well capable to benefit others
- One is able to get past the superficial level of information and recognise the intent
- One builds up knowledge, tolerance and understanding
- One can now make rational decisions
- One can prepare remedy to conflict and complications
- One becomes more learned

They say (or they used to say) that something as light as the beating off a butterfly`s wing on one continent could trigger a hurricane on another. Nobody ever proved or disproved this.
Perhaps one could entertain the same hypotheses about patient listening; it can create hurricanes just through 1) its power to acknowledge what someone is saying is important and 2) by your silence and respect for their words however different or compliant.

Regret and dissatisfaction
Many of the worlds' top athletes are spurred on by dissatisfaction and regret. It is not such a bad thing, but one doesn't want to indulge it. Often the chance to atone defeat comes from the void regretting missing opportunities to train harder, longer even smarter and add

to that a whole host of extra encouragement in diet and lifestyle choices and a touch of regret and dissatisfaction doesn't sound so bad, does it? Simply put it allows us to analyse the past and the future and to understand connection:

Making a mistake can be a powerful learning opportunity. From all mistakes comes success or another mistake which inevitably leads to better thinking, better solutions, alternatives or construction. Often we may ask you 'How did I get myself into that? Why?' And there is always a tinge of regret and dissatisfaction in our choice. But we also have the choice to move onwards and that is the beauty of life. You can choose happiness by using that dissatisfaction or regret to propel us forward. For instance, something as simple as a reparative apology to a colleague to returned goods which we don't really need defining us as we seek solutions to our reason for doing this or that. Regrets and dissatisfaction help you to change (think of them as the falling leaf I talked about earlier) and further to this shows that you care about the aftermaths of your doings.

Happiness blockers come when we confuse dissatisfaction with incompetence. The immediate thoughts there conjure up images of also-ran or failure.

Have you ever seen the message on the computer that states, 'In order for this computer to safely start up you need to press the safe key' which as we know helps to restart the computer after error Often the Happiness blocker level rises to new heights especially when you are in the middle of an 'important' task? Confusion follow, and anxiety threatens as does anger; all the detractors of happiness when in large doses. And this appears a large dose, doesn't it?

When will the computer restart will it ever and if it does will all my work be saved?
So, you punch away on the tabs pressing a random selection of keys thinking you can reorganise what was imperative to function meanwhile the computer is off into its own merry land readjusting or CHANGING. You get nowhere, boredom ensues and perhaps introspection; reasons why your files needed to be deleted or replaced in the first place.

Life is like that. So how do we take positives out of this? If anything, the computer error has taught you a lesson – we all need to reboot every now and then to delete unnecessary files we have collected along the way and implement new ones.

Apparent happiness blockers born out of non-ideal situations realise satisfaction when we get the context of why it happens. In turn satisfaction realise happiness!

Despondency

Despondency goes by many synonyms such as sadness, sorrow, grief and blues and its chief side effect is change, and as a result, solutions. Often in situations where despondency occurs for instance where we may lose a loved or suddenly are faced with devastating news re work, relationships or attachments we try to make right the reason of our distress.

Despondency encourages change and encourages clarity. Get everything into perspective, a step by step programme or check list which aids adapting to the newly imposed or voluntary change. Out the door goes random chaotic thinking, vulnerability or acting loosely without a goal. At the same time fairness and a quick return to your default programme re values morals and boundaries arise without fanfare. It is the acceptance of despondency which makes think harder and detracts from happiness; the ability to confirm that this event has occurred to challenge your thinking and reasons.

Despondency has other factors attached to it which help change it to happiness. The empathy of others when they see you down, sad or in anguish highlights the emotive response in the human brain. And researchers have concluded that it is possible we don't have one single emotional centre but different emotion centres. In a 1995 article paraphrased from the science section in, 'the New York times', according to psychiatrist, Dr Mark George at the National Institute of mental health in Bethesda, despondency and happiness involve two distinct brain areas. Further to this, women differ from men in their centre functions. Sadness in a woman revealed according to testing an increase in 'activity in the limbic system near the face and increased activity in the left prefrontal cortex than in the right'. When subjects were happy there was notable decrease in the commotion of the cerebral cortex correlated to organization and pre-thought (these areas are just above and behind the ears and just behind the forehead.)'

So there appears an interrelationship within systems which tag team one another in times of happiness and sadness.

When others see and feel our sadness and happiness perhaps they too will connect either directly or indirectly invoking change in these very same systems which acts as a contagion uplifting communal spirit helping both the despondent and helper to cope and move forward.

Further to this evading despondency or resentment, confusion or boredom, removing ourselves from those emotions that invoke hurt and change in mood doesn't serve us to grow and mature in fact it inhibits our effective running systems in mind body and spirit; in short it stunts personal and growth. It stops us from accepting that with happiness goes hurt and that we are constantly changing in order to reboot and understand where our priorities lay

History is being rewritten all day, every day. We all think that somehow, we are entitled to look back at various events and read into them, more than anyone saw at the time.

Keep pushing forward - Onwards and upwards. People care. We all go through similar challenges. Realize that self-pity is not helpful. Happiness is not about feeling sorry for yourself. It's about forgiveness, acceptance and we can do that by taking the time to analyse and explain.

'Remember rainbows only appear near a black cloud' – Michael Father Senior

11. Greatness Ahead – **look OUT!**

Nowadays, greatness gets lost in the wash of materialism and narcissism and so to happiness which becomes blurred in its definition, yet the United Nations considered the latter's impact so forceful that it 'designated' 20th March the International Day of Happiness. In 2012 there was even commissioned a World Happiness Report. The debate continues in earnest about the influence religion, spiritual and social cues including how much impact fear and finances and other mind, body and spirit factors play a role in determining its power. So, you see there is much ado about happiness

One thing is for sure amongst all the research there is no denying Happiness however long it lasts is still too short for worry. It is too short, too, for mistrust. And happiness is surely too short for investing hours in making long lists of all the things that it is too short for. Sometimes, if we are not careful, we create the very problems we declare ourselves to be most determined to avoid. We create the unhappiness.

Society is spellbound by the notion of winners and losers; victory and defeat. It's the thing that sells newspapers and fills social media. Therein lays one of the reasons we have such a competitive nation, underpinned by one upmanship and perceived admiration. Again, it is another reason why currently we are so obsessed with sport, cooking shows, *Survivor, Big brother, I'm a celebrity get me out of here* and game shows. Basically, we want to know, who is going to be a winner or a loser today/this month/this year/' and who will perceive to be happy or sad as a result. Why? We almost are conditioned to believe they are the only instincts that equate to winners and losers'.
Happiness`s battles are not 'won' and 'lost' moment by moment. We lose when we give way to what we believe we CANNOT change.

8 HAPPINESS Scientific FACTS to Change the Way you live now!

1. Studies at the University of Pennsylvania, in the effect of gratitude in 2005 confirmed what most of us already know, 'One of the greatest contributing factors to overall happiness in life is how much gratitude we show. 'I appreciate that', 'That is great, 'I'm so grateful' and a simple 'Thankyou' can be enough to convey our many thanks.

2. Lessons at the Claremont Graduate University, 2011 revealed that 3 simple things play a role in exciting the brains neurons to invite happiness. 1) Belief, 2) understanding, and 3) ethics increase as their levels of the brain's wonder drug ,oxytocin, increase.

Oxytocin is the drug mothers feeling with their new born and the very same drug which ignites when we receive or give a hug. Hint. Hint.

3. Make a good day great... Smile. Research at Michigan State University in 2011 suggested recalling happy events past has been found to encourage smiling this smiling has been found to be contagious especially when done at someone else. Think about any time you have been to a party and the smiles flow. It is very rare to find a gloom and doom soldier amongst a bunch of smiles. Now recall some fun times and the smiles start again and what do you feel? Yep, happy!

4. In one significant study at University of California, San Diego, in 2008 aptly named, The Dynamic Spread of Happiness, research suggested gathering amongst likeminded happy people 'rubbed off' on one's persona and encouraged a healthy happy attitude post days, weeks, months and years.

5. The 75-year wide Grant and Glueck research led by George Valiant and Sheldon Glueck arguably established happiness is not found by heated competition and enemies, but 'good relationships keep us happier and healthier'.

6. At the University of British Columbia, 2012, students at a certain rudimentary school whose deeds were for the benefit of others were more at ease and appreciated amongst their fellow students. 'Give and you shall receive' and this more than confirms the benefit of a kind act.

7. Money winnings create short term happiness only. Happiness fades quickly after a win in the lottery or gambling substitutes. People who have won the money appear no happier than those who haven't.

8. Create a moment. Research indicates people who spend time together just for 10 minutes a day hold happiness together longer than any new toy, home or car. The family that stays together becomes happy together and remember that applies to extended family and friends. Get to the zoo, take a picnic, play aboard game, read together, go to the park or garden.

12. MY LIST of Greatness Ingredients
Greatness starts NOW

1. Add a pinch of 'Director': I walk my own path that is I am responsible for what I do and where I go;

2. Grab a handful of thoughts: Where my mind goes my future follows;

3. Add a handful of the Present- Now is the start of action;

4. Remove - any excess Guilt: Everyone, at some stage of their life, wears self-guilt – you just don't want it to be a comfortable fit;

5. Sprinkle - some Hopes: Thoughts create action and thoughts are just that – ready to be turned over in my mind and if need be replaced with better ones;

6. Garnish - with Creation: I create angst and apprehension; I create joy and confidence;

7. Prepare - Change: Life is ever-changing courtesy of those who change it – a difference to others and to myself;

8. Beware - of overcooking: Perfection: The world isn`t perfect because I am not;

9. Watch and listen - Re birth: I have a chance to be new like each dawning day, pristine, embodied by good deeds done and good words spoken;

10. Care - Impact: The day that was yesterday impacts on this day and tomorrow if I choose to let it;

11. Share or OWE: I give my time and help others;

12. Sprinkle with Empathy: Listen to others to understand them;

13. Imbue - Strength: I am here and my reason for being here is I am a good person looking to embrace challenge that rewards me with awareness, understanding, acceptance and respect and love. My strength is all this.

'If one listens one will hear
If one looks, one will see,
If one touches one will feel
If one tries one will be.'
- anonymous

Bonus section:
*Loving Yourself?

When Frank Sinatra sang 'When you love somebody it's no good unless they love you all the way...' he was perhaps being melodic about the love essential to have for ourselves.

Not knowing how to love yourself is the permanent imbedded thorn in the side of the crown perched where all thought is processed – the mind. Feel like you've got no rhythm? Do you keep losing yourself? It is a nagging almost piercing yet stubborn injustice, discomfort and self-denial of the most wondrous thing in the world to deny loving yourself.

The most violent of all wars is the perpetual one which wages within your mind. As long as it continues your right to live happily will fluctuate wildly within the confines of those limbic and prefrontal cortex centres proposed earlier.

Furthermore, the angst you propose for yourself and encourage through thought and action will attract others to you like iron filings to a magnet. And the truth be said the converse is true i.e. love and happiness will attract love and happiness. So, in order for you to experience happiness, you need to know how to love yourself first and be happy then your rewards will follow.

It was Carl Jung who said, 'Who looks outside, dreams; who looks inside awakes.'
Invite the love and accept that others will complement and ignite this love.
When we seek to be above the pack to be above and beyond others ignoring the ingredients of happiness we are effectively looking outside. We start to become disconnected from all the happiness we deserve. To truly know love and happiness, we just need to become aware, look inside, and understand that we are not just a separate part we are part of the flowing wind that rushes from one side of the globe to the next; ebbing and flowing with conditions. Ideally, we are not a single entity seeking happiness rather part of a whole; each gust of wind and energy behind and with it working together to create change.

To fiddle around with a William Shakespeare quote, *We, all feel like the world is a stage and we are merely players.* Ah, if only life was as unassuming as performing take after take, and having an editor on standby to crop out the bits that seek to compromise us; to see where we could edit our life? But if we could, would we?

Markedly we are distinct by our life journey and how we respond and act upon requests and challenges, judgments and misfortunes, accomplishments and downfalls. Often, we believe that our fate has been, calculated; the path we take predestined and there is nothing we can do about it. Yet nothing could be further from the truth. In fact, when we entertain fate and destiny we should entertain bigger notions; ones that celebrate our bravery, integrity and love; love for our self.

Time and again the most successful person to uphold is the regular everyday person. You see the everyday person has to own their mistakes, invite patience, battle ignorance fight fear with the ambiguity that comes with each day without fanfare or bouquets.

These times we feel almost a duty to strive for perfection and merit. And it is in the process preconceiving what we do and achieve materialistically as happiness therewith evaporates into a smelly gas as we realise they are values misplaced and championed from another standpoint; with hands in pockets reaching for recompense for things we thought mattered. And we have all succumbed to temptation and we all fail, misunderstand and make mistakes. It has happened, does happen and will happen.

Compelling ownership of failure, misunderstanding and mistakes and learning to speak and act from it, at the same time as eluding the impulse to punch at the conceivable pre-conditioned shining default control to conceal our innermost feelings is a frank and honest emotion. There is no shame nor embarrassment in this. It is called loving yourself.

To love yourself doesn't mean engrossing a self-image obsessed disposition. It is not narcissism nor is it a medal to pin upon a puffed chest.

You love yourself in countless brave and egoless ways and means:

- To reconnect with the beauty of life after physical, mental and even spiritual sickness and ailment is to love yourself;

- To invite love and forgiveness after being left or abandoned as a child, friend, spouse or lover is to love yourself;

- To move forwards adapting to change after bereavement is to love yourself;

- To walk your way with mental and physical difficulties is to love yourself;

- To be true to you resisting temptation and ego driven rewards is to love yourself;

- To uphold beliefs and values in the face of adversity is to love yourself;

- To battle fear and ignorance, vexations to the spirit, is to love yourself.

Everyone at some time has felt the struggle to feel accepted and for many the feeling is stubborn almost unbreakable. We strive to do our best but the link to love and happiness is sometimes bent even broken. Every now and then as an upshot we don`t do our finest work.

One motive for not always doing our best is because sometimes, we imagine the gods are against us; the universe has another path set aside for us. Accordingly, we sense an innate attachment to those things we feel we deserve namely impatience, anxiety and even animosity. We don`t love ourselves the way or in the volume we should to see the constructive optimistic happy way forward. Following on from this is the idea what ensued was just desserts i.e. we be worthy of it. Now almost as a given the failure mentality comes out to play that person who seeks sadness and disappointment over happiness. You've seen it perhaps felt it, even said it, 'why does it always happen to me'. And hence forth, battle weary, one's contribution becomes unenthusiastic and almost purposeless. And look out friends and family and loved ones you will be the scorn of the developed derision.

People see love and happiness as being too abridge too far like the pot of gold at the end of the rainbow that only the leaping leprechaun's hold. Perhaps the leprechaun juggled some uncertainty whilst clearing a range of obstacles to get to the gold - we may never know yet their work may very well go unnoticed for the mere mortal. The work needed to bring our pot of gold or love happiness into our life is seen as something for 'Tomorrow' and almost too nobly in its passage. Add to this many philosophers or religious scribes and their bellowing from the soapbox, 'Happiness will start on judgement day and judgement day is coming and henceforth eternal Happiness. If not look out eternal hell!' and you create the all too hard basket.

But take note love and happiness is already here. One just doesn't know how to safely remove those obstacles on the nobly path to the pot of gold.

And what are those obstacles?

1. Greed
2. Self-centredness and
3. Egotism

Repeatedly we may wait a while for love and happiness to come knocking, whilst it waits for us to come to it. Often shame cements our footsteps to the nobly ground and a feeling of unworthiness or guilt yet we all can celebrate kind-heartedness, compassion and goodness in ourselves – we all have it - just look at our daily do's in thoughts, words and actions. True love and happiness doesn't warrant admiration or acknowledgement in the interim.

So where is your love and happiness?
They are in your thoughts, words and actions.

And to prove this ask yourself these 5 questions and I bet every one of them will answered differently to what you thought love and happiness for yourself warranted.

1. What would you do if you were told you had 2 weeks to live?
2. How would you mend broken friendships and relationships?
3. How would you help your family in sorrow?
4. What would you tell someone when you are about to leave this world?
5. How would you make someone smile?

Your answers would probably contain no materialistic choices. In fact, most of these answers would be underpinned by your true values; who you truly are. You have loved yourself for who you really are-and for this there is no greater Happiness.

'No one can truly love us like ourselves. No one can, and no one will. We must feel the love and only then does happiness extend its hand.'
– Michael

Conclusion

If at first you questioned *the Secret Recipe to Feeling Great* INSTANTLY you may have pretended all sorts of existentialism in tandem with the pursuit for piousness. You may have debated the merits of many things outside and aside from what has been discussed. But make no mistake, life is an endless practice in self-development. The happiness attached to the greatness treads a meandering curve that begins at birth and never ceases until the final breath. Whilst the initial development stems around one's schooling, hobbies, family, friends and employment sometimes an over-zealous ambition, self-centredness and ego places our happiness and life in a detour which with proper recognition returns us to where it is we deserve to be.

The Secret Recipe to Feeling Great INSTANTLY has as its mainstay ingredients of sorts: The existence of social, moral, family and employment values, ethics, moral and / or social compass, thankfulness, and perhaps the existence and conception of greater power or deity. It also lends itself to scientific study and even atheism. It has as its main ingredients that which seeks to invite you into a simplistic courteous way of life.

Make no mistake the meaning of feeling great is underpinned by our happiness which is one of the ultimate quests among many who seek to challenge their right to it. But you can be happier, starting right now, with small, purposeful steps open to everyone. We have delved into the wisdom of the ages, current academic study, and instructions from popular principles about how to be happier; the many challenges ensuring we are amongst the powerful sources of happiness.

Perhaps you will take it upon yourself and create your own recipe to feeling great. If mine took a leaf to fall from a tree to make me change then what will it take for you?

Other Books by Michael Guidner

- **Softly, Softly Catchee Monkey**

10 EASY CONFIDENCE 'TRICKS' To Take YOU to the TOP of the MOUNTAIN!
Work, home, relationships and love. Easy and simple if you know how!

- **The Secret Recipe for BEAUTIFUL**

Inside to Out. Lovely Pretty Gorgeous. For Women ONLY!

- **The SECRET Recipe for PERFECT POSTURE**

Revealed at LAST! How from years of research I found All the INGREDIENTS to: Banish the headaches, relieve back pain, stop the tiredness, change the hunchback, create and maintain the Perfect Posture!

- **The Secret RECIPE to FEELING Great INSTANTLY!**

Revealed at LAST! How I found All the INGREDIENTS to: Forgive the Past, look forward to tomorrow, and smile like a split watermelon

About the Author

Michael Guidner is an author, health analyst and motivational instructor. He is a talented writer and his edgy, inspiring, motivational and educational tips and techniques help to develop your own ideas and values towards becoming the best person you can and deserve to be!

References and Further Reading:

22 Encarta Dictionary English

Carlson R. You Can be happy, new world Library, 2010

Chaitow L. Stress, Harper Collins, 1983

Chodron P. When Things Fall Apart, Shambhala Publications, 1997

Chopra D. Self Power, Rider Books, 2012

Chopra D. The 7 Spiritual Laws of Success, New World Library, 1994

Chopra D. Ageless Body Timeless Mind, Rider Books, 2008

Carnegie D. How to Stop Worrying and Start Living, Richard Clay ltd, 1948

Carnegie D. How to win friends and Influence people, 1949

Day. J, LONELINESS-Don't feel like a prisoner in your own life! Set yourself free, Amazon, 2017

Day. J, 365 INSTANT LIFE CHANGING HABITS to achieve your dreams and wishes! Solve Life's Problems, Amazon, 2017

Day. J, SWING ON A STAR, Worry anxiety stress fear shame defeat Vs Peace happiness motivation success love victory, Amazon 2017

Guidner. M, The Secret Recipe for BEAUTIFUL. For Women ONLY! Amazon, 2017

Guidner. M, The Secret Recipe for Perfect Posture, Amazon, 2017

Pease A and B. The Definitive Book of Body Language, Manjul Publishing House, 2004

Senior, M. F. WHERE DID MY STRESS GO? Serenity One, Amazon, 2014

Senior, Michael Father. HOW TO Bring Back HAPPY into Your Life! Serenity One, Amazon, 2014

Senior, Michael Father. HOW to be the Best Person You Can Be, Serenity One, Amazon, 2014

Senior, Michael Father. The 5 Secrets of CONFIDENCE: Powerful Methods in Personal Change, Serenity One, Amazon, 2014

Senior, Michael Father. HOW to SURVIVE the DEATH of a LOVED One, Serenity One, Amazon, 2014

Senior, Michael Father. HOW to Farewell a Loved One, Serenity One, Amazon, 2014

Shoemaker Bill W. Alcoholics Anonymous, Isbn 1-893000716-2 1939

Smiles S. Self Help, Public Domain, 1859

Wholey D. The Miracle of Change, Simon And Schuster, 1997

Mn Mead Benefit of Sunlight, ncbi.nlm.nih.gov, 2008

Other
Healthdirect.gov.au

Wikipedia

Ncbi.nlm.nih.gov

Mindfulness.org

Psychology Australia

Notes:
* According to Dolores Hayden's article in California History, Mason's great-granddaughter Gladys Owens Smith quoted Mason as saying,

22 Encarta Dictionary English

Henricks, T. (2012). Selves, societies, and emotions: Understanding the pathways of experience. Boulder, Co: Paradigm.

James, H. (1956). The Bostonians: A novel. New York: Modern Library, p. 162.

www.ingramcontent.com/pod-product-compliance
Lightning Source LLC
Chambersburg PA
CBHW082214220526
45470CB00010B/3161